Angina

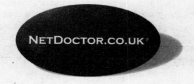

Series Editor
Dr Dan Rutherford

Hodder & Stoughton
LONDON SYDNEY AUCKLAND

Copyright © 2002 by NetDoctor.co.uk
Illustrations copyright © 2002 by Amanda Williams

First published in Great Britain in 2002

The right of NetDoctor.co.uk to be identified as the Author
of the Work has been asserted by them in accordance
with the Copyright, Designs and Patents Act 1988.

10 9 8 7 6 5 4 3 2 1

British Library Cataloguing in Publication Data
A record for this book is available from the British Library

ISBN 0 340 78685 X

Typeset by Avon Dataset Ltd, Bidford-on-Avon, Warks

Printed and bound in Great Britain by
Bookmarque

Hodder & Stoughton
A Division of Hodder Headline Ltd
338 Euston Road
London NW1 3BH
www.madaboutbooks.com

Contents

Foreword

Chest pain is a great source of anxiety to patients and doctors alike. This is because the pain may be angina. Angina is a pain that comes from the heart when there is an insufficient blood supply for the heart's needs. The usual cause for this is hardening of the heart arteries or coronary heart disease (CHD). CHD is the commonest single cause of death in the United Kingdom. However, if CHD is identified early and managed appropriately, it should be possible to reverse this terrible statistic.

This book sets out to explain in simple terms what is involved in this process and clearly describes all aspects of care from presentation to investigation, diagnosis and treatment. It emphasises the importance of not ignoring chest pain and of seeking advice quickly. It highlights the basic investigations that you should expect to help decide whether or not chest pain is anginal in nature. Equally importantly, an emphasis on prompt access to investigations in hospital where appropriate is stressed.

Once a diagnosis of angina has been made the book is upbeat in describing what is possible to treat the condition to improve the quality and quantity of life. The drugs used to treat CHD are clearly described as are more complex interventional treatments such as angioplasty and coronary artery bypass grafting. Equal emphasis is placed on what is possible for the patient to do to help themselves.

This book should enable the patient with angina to understand the condition but also to know what should be done. There are now clear standards being set by Government to ensure that we improve the management of CHD. We can meet those standards and go on to do even better. The best way to do this is for doctors, nurses and patients to work in partnership with a greater understanding of the illness. This book allows the patient to enter into the partnership fully motivated and well informed. I hope that it will be widely read.

Dr Mark Francis MA (Oxon), D.Phil, FRCP Edin
Consultant Cardiologist
Victoria Hospital
Kirkcaldy

Acknowledgements

Several people have been invaluable in producing this book, notably Dr Mark Francis, consultant cardiologist at Victoria Hospital, Kirkcaldy, Fife. Heart specialists are among the hardest pressed of all health professionals and I thank him sincerely for showing no hesitation in agreeing to review the material presented here.

Linda Walker and Anne McEwan, from the cardiovascular service in Dunfermline and West Fife, developed the excellent information pack for health personnel that was a useful resource in writing the book. Thanks are also due to Nicola Lee for checking the dietary information.

Judith Longman and Julie Hatherall at Hodder & Stoughton continue to absorb the departures from deadlines with a cheerful professionalism that is both admired and appreciated.

Great care is taken to ensure the accuracy of the NetDoctor book series and the responsibility for any errors is mine. Please let me know if you spot any, or if you have any suggestions concerning these books. I can be contacted at d.rutherford@netdoctor.co.uk

Dr Dan Rutherford
Medical Director
www.netdoctor.co.uk

Chapter 1

What is Angina?

'Angina' is one of those medical words that are used so often they are now part of ordinary language. The term comes from the Latin, meaning a 'spasm of the chest', and has similar roots to the word 'anguish'. In Greek and old French the equivalent word means strangling or choking. To many people who have angina these will be accurate words to describe how they feel during an attack.

Angina occurs when the blood supply getting to the muscle of the heart is insufficient for the amount of work the heart needs to do. The heart needs a lot of oxygen when it is working hard, during exercise for example, and less when it is at rest, so angina usually comes and goes depending on what a person is doing at any point in time.

The first description of angina is usually credited to an eighteenth-century physician, William Heberden, in a paper published in 1772 (although an Italian, Giovanni Morgagni, also described the condition convincingly several years earlier). Heberden said:

> There is a disorder of the breast marked with strong and peculiar symptoms, considerable for the . . . sense of strangling and anxiety with which it is attended . . . They are seized while they are walking (more especially if it be up a hill and soon after eating) with a painful and most disagreeable sensation in the breast . . . but the moment they stand still, all this uneasiness vanishes.

Angina (sometimes more fully called angina pectoris) is not a disease in itself but is a symptom of other diseases. By far the commonest cause of angina is narrowing of the arteries that take blood to the heart muscle – called the coronary arteries. So important is this single issue, called coronary artery disease or coronary heart disease (CHD), that a whole area of medical and scientific research is devoted to finding its causes and treatments. There are other conditions that can cause angina, such as when there is a tight heart valve putting an excessive load upon the heart, and we will also cover these in the book, but in terms of the numbers of people affected CHD is easily the commonest cause of angina.

The size of the problem

Angina affects over 1.5 million people in the UK, or about 10 per cent of the adult population in the middle or later age groups. In severity it can be very mild, or markedly disabling, or somewhere in between. The worst outcome for someone with CHD is that they go on to have a heart attack – in which permanent heart muscle damage is caused by complete blockage of a part of the heart's blood supply. Over 270,000 people in the UK suffer a heart attack every year – one person every two minutes – and 30 per cent of those people die before they reach hospital. Sometimes a heart attack will be the first sign that CHD is present but it is commoner for angina to develop first. In the UK an estimated 125,000 people a year die from CHD – it is the commonest single cause of adult deaths once one has excluded all types of cancer.

CHD in different groups

Our track record for CHD in the UK is bad – our death rates are among the highest in the world. Even within the UK there are marked differences between geographical regions, socio-economic and ethnic groups.

CHD is more common in the north of Britain compared to the south, with Scotland and Northern Ireland the worst areas. The premature death rate for men living in Scotland is 50 per cent higher than for men in East Anglia and for women it is 80 per cent higher. Manual workers are worse off than non-manual workers, and this difference is also particularly noticeable in women.

People of southern Asian origin (India, Pakistan, Bangladesh, Sri Lanka) who live in the UK are more likely to have CHD than average.

There are multiple reasons for these observed differences and we don't yet know what they all are, but the trends in CHD are mirrored by behaviour that we do know is associated with increased risk of developing CHD. For example, 36 per cent of male manual workers smoke compared to 21 per cent of non-manual workers. South Asians are less likely than other ethnic groups to take regular exercise. People in northern Britain and in lower income groups eat less fresh fruit and vegetables. More details on risk factors for CHD, and what to do about them, follow later in the book.

Recent trends

Since the 1970s significant falls in the death rates from CHD have been observed in many countries, but we are only beginning to see such falls in the UK. The trend for non-fatal CHD is however the opposite – there are more people now suffering this condition than ever before. This suggests we are getting better at treating heart attacks when they occur but getting worse at stopping people joining the queue to have one in the first place.

The extent of the differences seen between different economic groups has increased in the past 20 years, yet the care available to more disadvantaged sections of the population is often worse than that provided in more affluent parts of the country.

These are facts that make for poor reading. Partially they reflect a general trend in western society for an increase in so-called 'lifestyle' diseases. Diabetes is another such condition that is rapidly on the increase and which has much in common with CHD in the types of risk factor associated with its cause, such as lack of exercise, obesity and poor diet.

Making improvements

The extent of the problem is well recognised but the level of medical care presently offered in the UK to sufferers of CHD is at best patchy and too often is inadequate. The government's desire to improve the prevention, detection and treatment of CHD is set out in the National Service Framework for the condition (see appendix A for details).

CHD is one of our biggest medical enemies. Tackling it is actually everyone's business – not just the health service personnel who deliver the medical care, or the politicians who decide our taxes and allocate the funding. A lot of the improvement needed in CHD will have to come from the actions we take as individuals and the way we all live our lives.

This book tries to explain angina and CHD in some detail. It should be useful to you if you have angina, or know someone who does, or if angina runs in your family. It will explain what you can do to help yourself if you have angina now or to reduce your chances of getting angina in the future. It will also explain the care you should expect to receive from a modern health service – the sorts of medicines and other treatments available and why and when they are used.

No one can deny that in Britain we have a lot of work to do to get CHD under control, and in many ways we have fallen behind other developed countries with similar problems. On the other hand many of the world's best specialists in heart disease live and work in Britain. Much of the effort that is needed in CHD is the same as is needed to control diabetes and high blood pressure – two of the other main public health problems we need to tackle. It will all take time, but now is always a good time to start.

Chapter 2

Structure of the Heart and Circulation

Understanding a bit about the structure of the heart and how it functions makes it a lot easier to follow what goes on in angina and why various types of treatment have been developed. Often the groundwork in any subject is the boring bit, and there is a temptation to skip through it, but in the case of the heart so much of it is amazing that you'll be tempted to read on!

The heart as a pump

The main function of the heart is of course to drive blood around the complex network of blood vessels that makes up our circulation. The heart of a foetus starts to beat on the twenty-second day following conception. A few days later the primitive circulation starts to flow, and the work of a lifetime is then well under way.

An adult's heart is a roughly cone-shaped organ slightly bigger in size than a clenched fist. It sits in the chest behind the breastbone, mostly in the middle but offset slightly to the left side (see figure 1). The heart is hollow and contains four chambers, and is made up almost entirely of muscle. When empty of blood an adult woman's heart weighs about 250 grams, a man's about 275 grams.

Figure 1: Position of the heart within the chest

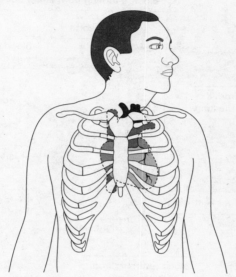

Strictly speaking the heart is two pumps that work together because, in common with other higher animals, man has a double circulation. One half of the heart – the right side – receives blood returning from the body and pumps it through the lungs, where the blood receives a fresh charge of oxygen and waste carbon dioxide is released to be breathed out. The left side of the heart receives this oxygen-rich blood from the lungs and pumps it out to the rest of the body, so continuing the cycle.

Each side of the heart has two chambers – blood comes in first to the smaller chamber, called the atrium, which then sends it on to the much more muscular and powerful ventricle. The right ventricle pumps blood to the lungs and the left ventricle pumps blood to the body. An 'inlet' valve between each atrium and ventricle and an 'outlet' valve at the exit of each ventricle keeps blood flowing in one way only around each circuit. This is illustrated in figure 2.

Figure 2: The twin circulation of blood to the lungs and to the body

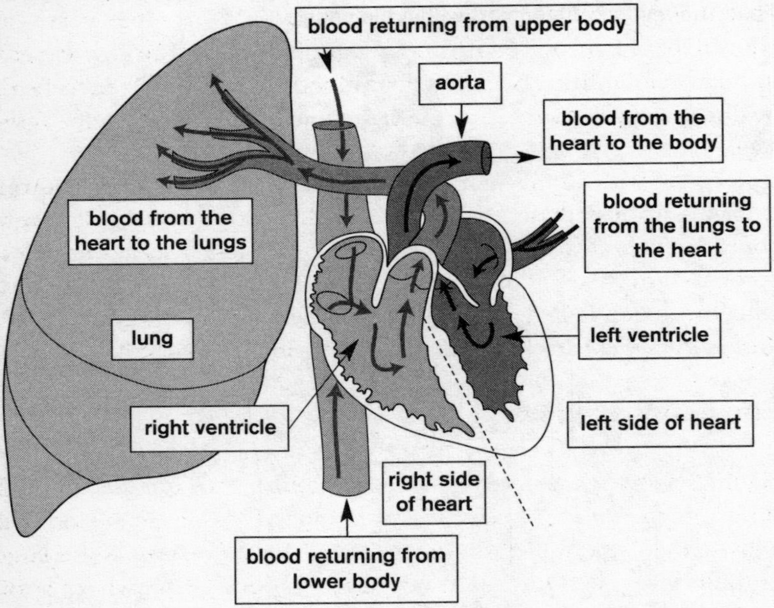

Each half of the heart works in synchronisation with the other, so both ventricles relax at the same time to fill up with blood and contract at the same time to pump blood out. The atria (plural of atrium) are fairly weak muscular chambers, which essentially help to fill the ventricles with blood prior to each heartbeat.

Because the amount of effort required to send blood around the body is much larger than that needed to push blood through the lungs, the muscle of the left ventricle is much thicker and stronger than that of the right. This also means that the left ventricle has a higher requirement for oxygen, and the consequences of poor blood supply to the muscle of the left ventricle are more serious than the same problem in the right ventricle. This is explained in more detail shortly when we consider the way the heart receives its blood.

Statistics about the heart's actions are quite impressive. Each beat of an adult heart puts out 70–80 millilitres (mls) of blood. There are about 70 beats per minute, so it pumps 5 litres of blood per minute. That makes 7,200 litres per day, or 2,628,000 litres per year – the equivalent of five swimming pools! During exercise, through increases in heart rate and in the amount of blood sent out with each beat, a healthy heart can increase its output to five times more than the resting state.

To cope with all this work, the heart uses a lot of energy. Although it makes up less than 0.5 per cent of the body's weight, it receives about 5 per cent of its own output of blood back to itself through the coronary arteries. These have the crucial job of supplying the heart with the required amount of oxygen and nutrients. Knowing about these arteries is central to understanding angina in detail.

Coronary arteries

Figure 3 shows the coronary arteries and how they are placed on the surface of the heart. The delivery of blood to the body is the job of the left ventricle, and the artery that receives this blood first is the largest in the body, called the aorta. At the base of the aorta, where it joins the heart, lies the aortic valve. This prevents blood that has just been pumped out from running back into the left ventricle. Immediately after the aortic valve there are two openings in the aorta, one on either side, which are the start of the left and right coronary arteries.

The right coronary artery runs down the right side of the heart, sending branches as it goes to the underlying heart muscle. The left coronary artery is more complex – it divides into two other main branches, which between them supply blood to the bulkier left ventricle, and to the muscular dividing wall (called the septum) that separates the right and left halves of the heart. It is worth knowing the names of these blood vessels as this subject comes up again later in

Figure 3: Position of the coronary arteries on the surface of the heart

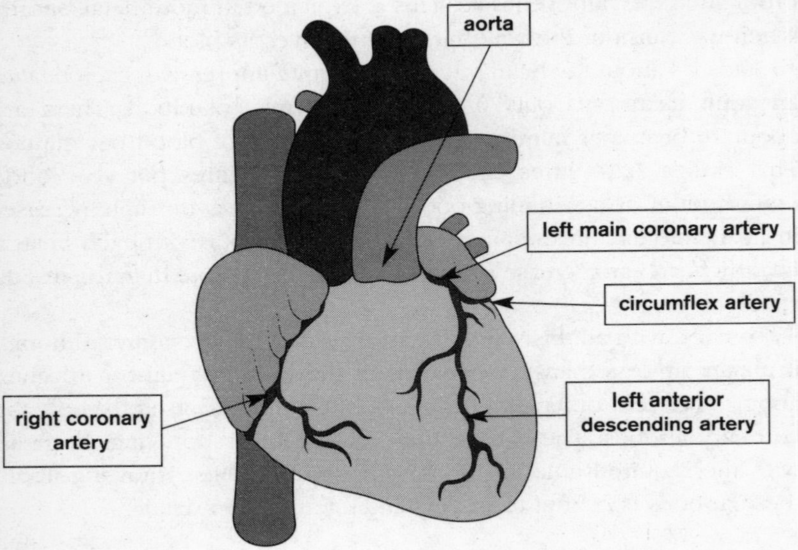

the book when we talk about bypass operations and angioplasty – the meaning of these terms will be explained when they arise.

The first part of the left coronary artery is called the left main coronary artery. Its branch that runs down the front of the heart is the left anterior descending artery ('anterior' is the medical word for 'front') and the other branch, which runs round the back of the heart, is called the circumflex artery.

In practical terms there are therefore three main arteries to the heart, although two of them come from one common origin. Each of them is the main source of blood to a large section of the heart muscle. Any one, two, or all three of these arteries can become blocked in the processes that cause coronary artery disease. Heart specialists (cardiologists) often refer to 'single, double or triple vessel disease' when discussing how many coronary arteries are involved in any individual troubled by angina. Variations in the exact way in which the arteries divide are quite common in human beings, but the basic layout is much the same in everyone. Disease within the left main or first part of the descending arteries is looked upon as a higher risk than disease elsewhere within the coronary artery system.

Oxygen demand

Heart muscle is greedy as far as oxygen is concerned. When blood flows through any area of the body a certain amount of oxygen is removed to satisfy the needs of that particular tissue or organ, then the blood flows through the veins back to the lungs to receive its next charge of oxygen. On average, most tissues and organs of the body extract only about 40 per cent of the oxygen that flows through them but the heart extracts 70 per cent even at rest. The need for oxygen may increase five-fold in times of heavy demand such as in strenuous exercise, so it becomes obvious how dependent the heart is upon a good supply of blood, and how limiting it can be when a partial blockage of one or more of these arteries develops.

The arteries of the body are muscular tubes, capable of narrowing or widening according to several controlling factors that we will touch upon later. The point is that the amount of blood flowing through the coronary arteries is not fixed but can vary up or down. Similarly we go through spells of rest and exercise when the heart's need for oxygen varies. It is only when there is an imbalance of these two factors (i.e. demand exceeding supply) that angina occurs. This is illustrated in figure 4. In the top part of the diagram the shaded area represents the ability of the coronary arteries to supply blood during the course of the day. In the lower half of the diagram the shaded area indicates the levels of demand of the heart for blood. Peaks would therefore represent bursts of exercise, for example. Where the two areas cross (shown as heavy shading) these are times when the amount of coronary blood flow is inadequate, and in a person these would be the times when angina is experienced.

One of the ways in which some drugs to treat angina work is by encouraging the coronary arteries to open wider, thus improving the blood flow to heart muscle.

Figure 4: The fluctuation in supply and demand on the heart over 24 hours

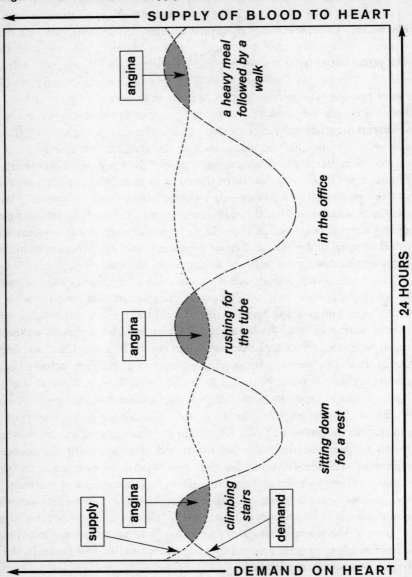

Coronary veins

Matching the network of coronary arteries is a system of veins that return blood that has passed through the heart muscle back to the 'input' side, where it joins the blood returning from the rest of the body. The veins of the heart, to all intents and purposes, do not give any trouble.

Coronary artery disease

It is clear that the heart is a remarkable piece of biological crafts-manship, but if it had been designed by a human engineer one can speculate that a few modifications might have been suggested. The coronary arteries are not huge vessels and they are fed blood from only two points of origin, yet they have to deliver a large volume of blood throughout life. Whereas the engine in a small aeroplane is made with a double set of spark plugs, we don't have a back-up system of arteries in the heart (or in other critical organs) that can take over if the first set becomes blocked. Extending the analogy a bit – if one of our plugs fails, we're in trouble.

Much research work has therefore been done to try to understand the reasons why arteries can become blocked. We don't yet fully understand the whole process, but many parts of the jigsaw have been worked out.

ATHEROSCLEROSIS

This is the medical term for the 'furring up' process that blocks arteries anywhere in the body. The alternative medical term is 'arteriosclerosis' and it means exactly the same thing.

If you took two arteries, one healthy and one affected by athero-sclerosis, cut them across and then inspected each under a microscope you would see something like that shown in figure 5. On the left is the normal artery, with a wide channel for the blood to flow through. The three layers of the artery are also labelled:

Figure 5: Healthy and diseased arteries

healthy artery

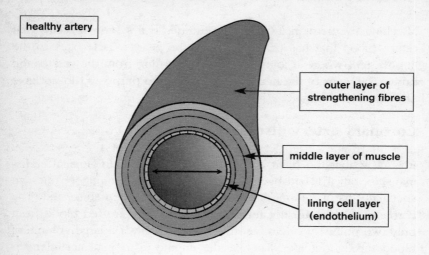

outer layer of strengthening fibres

middle layer of muscle

lining cell layer (endothelium)

diseased artery

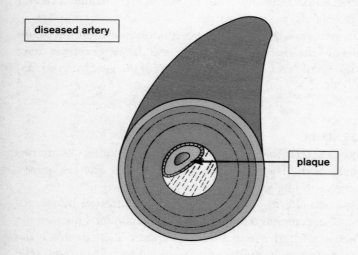

plaque

1   Lining (medical term is 'endothelium')
2   Middle layer of muscle
3   Outer layer of strengthening fibres

On the right is the diseased artery, substantially narrowed by thickening of the middle muscle layer and in particular by a fatty deposit that has built up under the endothelium. This is called plaque (and is nothing like the plaque that builds up on neglected teeth). The processes that cause plaque to form (and the methods of getting it to go away) are the central issues in coronary heart disease and in other conditions such as stroke, in which atherosclerosis is the main cause of the condition.

The lining of arteries (endothelium)

The thin layer of cells that lines all of our arteries has many important functions. These cells manufacture chemicals, the most important of which is nitric oxide, that cause the adjacent artery to either narrow or widen. When nitric oxide is released by these lining cells it has a powerful relaxing effect on the muscular layer of the artery which causes the artery to widen at that point.

Nitric oxide is formed when lightning zips through the atmosphere in a thunderstorm but in the body it is formed more sedately when oxygen is combined with an amino acid called L-arginine. The importance of nitric oxide within many vital chemical reactions that go on in the body was discovered only about 20 years ago and a huge amount of research has subsequently developed around it.

Nitric oxide appears to act upon artery lining in ways which prevent the changes of atherosclerosis from occurring. In people who have atherosclerosis the power of the lining cells to manufacture nitric oxide is reduced, not only in the diseased arteries but also in otherwise normal-looking arteries elsewhere in the body (it is common in atherosclerosis for diseased areas to be mixed in with apparently healthy arteries). It seems that a reduction in nitric oxide production is one of the early steps in the sequence of events that leads to atherosclerosis.

Disturbance in nitric oxide function is also seen in people who smoke, or have high blood pressure or raised amounts of cholesterol in the blood, so this appears to be one of the explanations for why people with these 'risk factors' are more likely to go on to develop CHD.

Plaque

Once the endothelial cells start to malfunction a number of other problems start to occur. First they attract the specialised scavenger cells of the immune system whose normal job it is to get rid of foreign invaders such as bacteria or dead tissue cells etc. These scavenger cells (called macrophages) then stick to areas of the endothelium and also build up just underneath it. Macrophages are good at latching on to certain types of fat that circulate in the blood – and so the build-up starts. At first there is just a thin layer of fats under the endothelium. With time this gets bigger, until sometimes it can build up so much that the capacity for the blood to get through is severely reduced. This is the common finding in someone who has angina. Fortunately the area affected by the narrowing is often fairly limited, which allows the doctor to treat the narrowed segment by, for example, stretching it open with specialised instruments. We shall come on to what exactly this means in chapter 7.

On top of causing an obstruction to blood flow, a plaque is also a weak point in an artery. In particular the thin covering of the plaque can rupture, exposing it and the underlying muscular artery layer. This can trigger another sequence of chemical reactions in the blood, which results in the blood clotting at the site of the plaque rupture. This is very often what occurs in a heart attack – suddenly what had been a narrowed artery can rapidly turn into a completely blocked one. If treated early enough with 'clot-busting' drugs this can limit or prevent lasting heart muscle damage (see chapter 6).

This occurrence of clotting within a coronary artery is now known to be extremely important. Older views of how heart attacks developed were constructed around the idea of an area of plaque gradually narrowing with time, slowly reducing the size of the gap within the coronary artery through which blood could flow. Ultimately the obstruction would become complete and blockage would occur. More recent research shows that the majority of heart attacks occur as a result of sudden blockage of arteries that do not have very tightly restricting areas of plaque. Instead the problem is that the plaque is unstable and more prone to surface breakdown and hence clot formation on top. These unstable plaques contain more cholesterol and are structurally weaker than an 'old' plaque containing more in the way of scar tissue. Old plaques are therefore less likely to suffer surface breakdown and lead on to a heart attack.

The importance of these points is two-fold. First, drugs which prevent clot forming in the first place (such as aspirin or clopidogrel – see chapter 6) will offer some protection against future heart attacks occurring. Second, drugs which reduce cholesterol will have beneficial effects by reducing the amount of plaque formation.

Further details about the role of cholesterol and other fats in coronary heart disease are to be found in chapter 4.

Chapter 3

Do I Have Angina?

If making a diagnosis of angina were straightforward, life would be a lot easier for many people – certainly for GPs and cardiologists but also for patients suffering, perhaps unknowingly, from the condition. In fact angina takes many forms and it can be a difficult job sorting it from the other conditions that can look like it. In this chapter we look at the sorts of features that point towards making an accurate diagnosis, starting with the symptoms that angina can cause and moving on to the initial sort of assessment your GP will be able to do. Later we look in more detail at the more complex investigations that are often needed in diagnosing and dealing with angina, and which require the help of a specialist in heart disease – a cardiologist.

Symptoms

There are many possible ways for angina to present itself and these ways can exist singly or in any combination. The main ones are:

- Discomfort, usually in the chest, which comes on with exertion or emotional upset and is relieved by rest.
- The commonest site of discomfort is behind the breast bone but other sites that can be affected include the left arm, right arm, throat, jaws, teeth or the back.
- The discomfort is often not described as a pain, but more as a tightness or constriction, a burning feeling, a dull ache or a sensation of feeling choked.
- Breathlessness on exertion, with or without pain.

The relationship of angina to exertion or stress is the main clue to the diagnosis in the first instance. Angina is usually due to a narrowing or blockage of the coronary arteries, so the symptoms mainly come on when the demand for blood is greater than can be temporarily supplied. Then, when the person rests, the amount of blood that can get through is enough for the resting heart. However, some people with angina, particularly when it is advanced, will get angina even at rest. Yet others get little or no chest pain but instead experience breathlessness on effort.

Severe angina can be accompanied by other symptoms such as sweating, anxiety and nausea, which are due to activity within the nervous system of the body brought on by the pain.

Angina can very easily seem like indigestion – the symptoms can be exactly the same in either case. Very few people have come to grief because of heartburn but many others who have mistakenly thought they had an upset stomach have turned out to have angina or a heart attack – sometimes with tragic results. This emphasises the need for any episode of severe chest pain to be taken seriously and why 'indigestion' needs to be suspected as angina in disguise, until proven otherwise.

WHY CAN ANGINA BE FELT IN DIFFERENT PARTS OF THE BODY?

A common cause of confusion is the fact that pain arising in the heart does not have to be felt directly where the heart is situated in the chest. The reason for this goes back to our development in the womb.

The heart develops very early in the embryo and is pumping by the fourth week. The cells that eventually form the heart arise from tissues that in the embryo at this stage are next door to each other and are located at the level of the upper neck. At the same time as these tissues are growing, so are the nerves which connect them to the spinal cord and brain of the embryo. Later, as the embryo enlarges, some of the structures that were located in the neck migrate down to take up their final position lower in the chest. The heart is one of the structures that do this. However, the nerve connections to the brain simply lengthen to make this possible – and as far as the brain is concerned the heart remains in the neck forever!

The brain is unable to distinguish exactly where pain is coming from if it arises from any of the tissues that were originally related in this same way. This is why the left arm as well as the other sites mentioned above can all be where the person who has it perceives heart pain – and it's important for doctors and patients not to be fooled by this.

If you get any symptoms that look remotely like these, or are in any doubt about your medical condition, always discuss how you feel with your doctor.

WHAT ELSE CAN CAUSE CHEST PAIN?

The possibilities are many. Here are some:

- Digestive system
  a) Acid reflux from the stomach into the lower gullet
  b) Spasm of the gullet
  c) Stomach or duodenal ulcer
  d) Gallstones

- Lungs
  a) Irritation of the lining of the chest cavity and surface of the lungs ('pleurisy')
  b) Tumour of the lung
  c) Clots in the lungs

- Bones and muscles
  a) Rib injury or inflammation
  b) Arthritis of the spine and neck

This is far from a complete list, but it illustrates the potential difficulty in diagnosing angina and why it can be necessary to carry out many other investigations to be sure.

Having said that, it is often possible for a doctor to be confident right away that angina is present. This will be when the person has a typical history of the right sort of discomfort on effort, relieved by rest. The likelihood of angina being present is increased if the person has other 'risk factors' for the development of coronary heart disease. These include:

- Older age group
- Male sex
- Cigarette smoking
- High blood pressure
- High blood cholesterol
- Family history of coronary heart disease
- Diabetes
- Obesity

Evidence of 'hardening of the arteries' (atherosclerosis) elsewhere in the body makes it more likely that coronary artery disease has also developed.

OTHER POSSIBILITIES

Rare heart problems

We'll come on to what happens in the course of examining and investigating someone with angina but important things that the doctor looks for at the start include evidence of tightness of the aortic heart valve. This is a fairly rare condition in general but a bit less so in the elderly, whose heart valves tend to thicken and become less flexible with age. A tight aortic valve can dramatically increase the amount of effort needed from the left ventricle to get blood out into the circulation, which in turn increases the demand of the ventricle muscle for oxygen. This can cause angina even if the coronary arteries are normal, because angina really represents a state when there is an imbalance between the demand and supply of the heart muscle for blood – whatever the cause. 'Stenosis' is the proper medical term for abnormal narrowing of a tube or opening in the body, so this condition where the main valve is tight is called aortic stenosis.

A rare condition exists in which the heart muscle over-develops and becomes very much thicker than normal. Because there is more heart muscle needing to be supplied with blood this can lead to demand outstripping supply once again, causing angina. The situation is made worse if the thickened muscle also causes narrowing of the left ventricle below the aortic valve, leading to a similar problem as occurs with a tight valve. This condition is called hypertrophic cardiomyopathy, or hypertrophic obstructive cardiomyopathy – HOCM (*hyper* = excessive, *trophic* = to do with growth or nourishment, *cardio* = to do with the heart, *myopathy* = any muscle disease).

High blood pressure

High blood pressure puts a similar strain on the heart but as high blood pressure is also a risk factor for developing hardening of the arteries in general it is also more likely that the coronary arteries in someone with high blood pressure will be narrowed. Effective treatment to lower the blood pressure will, however, reduce the load on the heart and may thereby relieve the angina.

Anaemia

Someone who is very anaemic ('bloodless') for whatever reason will, by definition, have fewer red cells in their blood. Red blood cells have the job of delivering oxygen, so it is possible for someone who is anaemic to develop angina. Usually such a person will also have narrowing of the coronary arteries although this might not have been apparent until the anaemia occurs, thus revealing the inadequacy of the heart's blood supply.

The doctor's assessment

When someone goes to the doctor for the first time with pains in the chest, or breathlessness, or these other symptoms we have just mentioned, the doctor has to narrow down the possible causes until the correct one is found.

AGE

The first useful piece of information is the age of the patient. Angina largely affects people in middle age or later, mainly because CHD affects that age group too. It is certainly possible for a young person (below 40) to have angina, but it is uncommon, and it is then more likely to be due to problems other than coronary artery disease or to be associated with conditions that cause premature coronary artery disease. One example is a hereditary condition in which affected family members have very high cholesterol levels in the blood, but the most common factor among people who develop coronary artery disease at a young age is that they almost always are smokers.

HISTORY

There should be lots of clues in the person's history that will point to or away from a likely diagnosis of angina. Angina comes on while there is increased demand on the heart – not afterwards – and is relieved by rest. So it comes on during exercise, or climbing stairs, or walking up a slope, etc. Cold weather and strong winds add to the effort of walking and are often noted by people with angina to be the times when they are at their worst. Emotional upset or excitement is another form of stress, so angina might relate to becoming angry or when excited watching a football match, for example. As we've seen, the exact site in the body of angina discomfort can be misleading, so if any of these suggestive symptoms seems to be related to effort or stress then angina should be suspected.

When we eat the body naturally diverts blood to the digestive system and away from everything else, including the heart. Angina is therefore sometimes more noticeable after a heavy meal. Going for a brisk walk after a large lunch on a windy winter's day is not the best idea for someone with bad angina. It would be better to wait an hour or two for the digestive process to have settled a bit and then to set a modest pace.

A frequent cause of difficulty in initial diagnosis comes from the fact that discomfort from the lower end of the gullet – the food tube connecting the throat to the stomach – can feel exactly like angina, right down to the radiation of the pain to the left arm and elsewhere. This harks back to the closeness of the heart and stomach in the early development of the human embryo and the difficulty the brain has in distinguishing pain from these structures. However, if someone with this pain also says that it is completely abolished by a couple of teaspoons of antacid mixture, it is a fair bet that they are not describing angina.

There are many other pointers from the history that can prove helpful, such as the fact that it is unusual for angina to be felt over the left side of the chest – where most people take the heart to be situated. Pains in this location are a fairly common cause of concern to healthy people in their 20s and 30s and are often due to inflammation of the ribs and muscles. Heart pains tend not to result in a catch in one's breathing on a deep breath – lung and rib or muscle problems are more likely to be the cause of that sort of pain. Heart pain tends to be prolonged, so chest pains lasting just a second or two are not likely to be from the heart.

Using such a system of probabilities the doctor can often narrow down the likely cause of chest pains. Going further to make a completely accurate diagnosis will then usually mean doing further tests, which are covered in the next chapter. It hopefully goes without saying that you should never try to make your own diagnosis of what is causing your chest pain, or any other important symptom. It is never a waste of a doctor's time to consult about chest pains. If they turn out to be due to some harmless cause, then well and good. Every doctor likes to be able to reassure someone that they have nothing to worry about!

VARIATIONS ON THE THEME

Everyone is different, and the exact way in which angina affects people can vary to quite a large degree. There are also many traps for the unwary in the field of chest pain in general. For example, you can get painless angina; you can get angina which does *not* need to be related to effort – it can occur when doing nothing; many a person thought to have 'indigestion' actually has severe angina, or a heart attack. A wise doctor will be reluctant to say categorically that angina is *not* present until further tests have been done in most patients. The upshot is that a lot of people with perfectly normal hearts need to be checked out fully before they can be properly reassured and sometimes, despite everyone's best efforts, people with angina get labelled with another, incorrect diagnosis.

OTHER INFORMATION

Many other pieces of information are required to make a full assessment of angina, and what to do about it. Your doctor may already hold some of this information in your medical notes and other information will need to be assessed or updated.

The important factors that a doctor looks for are those that directly or indirectly influence cardiovascular risk:

- Raised blood pressure
- Smoking tobacco
- Raised blood fat level (cholesterol in particular)
- Presence of diabetes
- Family history of coronary heart disease
- Excess body weight
- Diet high in fat and low in fresh fruit and vegetables
- Low exercise levels
- Raised alcohol intake
- Presence or absence of artery disease elsewhere in the body
- Presence or absence of heart valve abnormality, anaemia or other relevant medical conditions

PHYSICAL EXAMINATION

In many people with angina the general type of physical examination that your doctor can do will in fact be quite normal. However, the sorts of things a doctor looks for on examining a patient with angina, particularly for the first time, include:

Eyes

A white ring around the edge of the iris (coloured part of the eye) can be due to raised fat levels in the blood.

Skin colour

Tar staining on the fingers indicates cigarette smoking. Pale skin might indicate a lack of blood (anaemia).

Blood pressure

This is a very important measurement as high blood pressure increases the strain on the heart and is a 'risk factor' for the development of hardening of the arteries. Blood pressure, and the problems associated with it, is fully covered in the companion book on high blood pressure in this series. The most important facts are presented in chapter 5. Although high blood pressure increases the risk of developing angina, you *can* get angina with perfectly *normal* blood pressure.

Examination of the heart

By this is meant the basic inspection of the chest and listening to the sounds of the heart valves in action. When there is a tight heart valve, for example, the left ventricle builds up muscle in its efforts to overcome the obstruction. Often a doctor can detect this enlargement of the heart by feeling a thrusting 'heave' of the left rib cage with each beat. A tight aortic valve also makes a characteristic harsh noise (murmur) due to turbulence of the blood as it squeezes through the narrowed valve, and this can easily be heard with a stethoscope when it is significant. Heart valve problems are only rarely a cause of angina. Usually this part of the examination is normal.

Examination of the blood vessels

Here the doctor is looking for evidence that hardening of the arteries already exists elsewhere in the body, which increases the likelihood that it has developed in the heart arteries. A common way to do this is to check for the strength of the pulse behind the ankle bone or on the top of the foot. A reduction, or absence, of these pulses is usually due to atherosclerosis. Another way is to listen with a stethoscope over the main arteries (carotid arteries) which are on either side of the front of the neck. If these contain significantly narrowed areas due to a build up of plaque then the blood flowing through them may do so with a 'whooshing' sound. This is known as a 'bruit' (pronounced broo-ee). Quite advanced atherosclerosis can, however, be present with no detectable abnormality in any of the pulses of the body.

These features are listed as examples to help you understand the purpose of the doctor's examination. Remember though that there is some truth in the phrase 'a little knowledge is a bad thing'. Don't try and make your own diagnosis, or get into a state of anxiety if you can't find your ankle pulse! It is not easy to pick up these 'clinical signs' correctly, so let your doctor do the assessment.

By the time you have related your symptoms and the doctor has quizzed you on other aspects of how you feel, gathered the background information mentioned above and examined you, then a lot of information will have been obtained. Even so, the cause of your symptoms might still not be clear. It will then be necessary to move on to other tests, most of which will require you to be seen by a specialist.

When the diagnosis of angina does seem likely at this stage, you should still be referred to a heart specialist. That way you will benefit from the diagnosis being confirmed and will be assessed for the most effective treatment that suits your particular circumstances. What this means will become clear during the course of the rest of this book.

The next step though, is to explain what are these further tests, and what they mean.

Chapter 4

Investigating Angina

Although a specialist is required for the more sophisticated tests, your GP can do some basic investigations that are still very helpful. Increasingly GPs are organising specific clinics for CHD. These are commonly run with the help of nurses attached to the surgery, either within the primary care team or seconded to the practice for a while to help with calling up and assessing people known to have CHD. Although the doctor needs to be involved in making the initial diagnosis of angina, a lot of the follow-up work can be done very well (or better!) by a nurse.

Blood tests

The main information that blood tests reveal, and that is relevant to angina, is:

PRESENCE OF ANAEMIA

In anaemia there are fewer red blood cells in the circulation, and therefore a lower level of circulating oxygen. There are many possible causes of anaemia, so this needs to be investigated in its own right. Someone who has angina revealed by being anaemic will still have some degree of coronary artery disease but if it is mild then correction of the anaemia may abolish the angina.

SUGAR (GLUCOSE) LEVEL

Raised blood glucose is the hallmark of diabetes. Diabetic people are at two to four times greater risk of developing coronary artery disease than the non-diabetic population. Good control of the blood glucose level through careful attention to the diabetes reduces the likelihood of such complications.

BLOOD FAT (LIPID) LEVELS

This is a particularly important subject and is worth understanding in some detail. There is a bit of medical jargon attached to the subject which can't be avoided but isn't too indigestible.

There are two main types of lipid (the more general term for fat) that circulate normally in the blood – cholesterol and triglyceride. The benefits of lowering cholesterol are well established whereas with triglyceride the situation is less clear cut, so we will concentrate on cholesterol.

Cholesterol

Cholesterol is an important substance used by the body in many ways. It is the biochemical starting point for manufacture of many of the body's natural steroid hormones and of vitamin D, which is essential for the control of calcium within the body. It is also an essential component of the membrane that forms the walls of individual cells in all tissues.

Contrary to what you might think from the amount of publicity that cholesterol gets, the amount that is present in our blood is to a large extent independent of how much is in our diet. That does not mean that dietary cholesterol intake is unimportant (it *is* important) but it does mean that there is a lot more to the cholesterol story than how many fried eggs we eat a week.

Eighty per cent of the cholesterol we have is produced by chemical processes within our own body – mostly by the liver. It is then transported from the liver via the bloodstream to other tissues. It travels not as cholesterol molecules floating in the blood but as minute packages of cholesterol mixed with large molecules called lipoproteins. Lipoproteins are themselves combinations of fats and proteins and they work in a similar way to the detergents we use to wash up dishes. Fats such as cholesterol (and triglyceride) do not dissolve well in the watery realm of the bloodstream, but become soluble when coated with lipoproteins, in just the same way that detergents make grease soluble in water.

Four main groups of lipoproteins exist, based mainly on their different sizes and density:

1 High density lipoproteins (HDL)
2 Low density lipoproteins (LDL)
3 Very low density lipoproteins (VLDL)
4 Chylomicrons

Each of these types of lipoprotein has a different function in the body. For example, chylomicrons are the form in which fats (as cholesterol and triglyceride) are absorbed from the digestive system and transported to the bloodstream. The essential information when considering CHD is that high density lipoprotein (HDL) mops up excess cholesterol in the body and returns it to the liver for re-processing, whereas low density lipoprotein (LDL) is the form in which cholesterol is taken from the liver to be deposited elsewhere in the body.

LDL is the form of cholesterol and triglyceride mixture that is favoured for take-up by the scavenger cells of the artery lining cells mentioned earlier. It now becomes obvious why it is that LDL is often referred to as 'bad cholesterol' – and why the more you have of it in your blood the more likely you are to develop CHD.

HDL, because it attaches to excess cholesterol anywhere and returns it to the liver, is therefore called 'good cholesterol' – and raised amounts of it give protection against CHD.

Men generally have higher levels of LDL compared to women. This is probably because of the protective effect of oestrogen, one of the female hormones. This difference falls and eventually disappears in women following the menopause. Exercise raises HDL levels, as does modest alcohol intake.

Figures to remember

A couple of specific figures are worth knowing in connection with cholesterol, as you should be aware of your own level whether or not you have angina. The units of measurement are 'millimoles per litre', usually abbreviated to mmol/litre. Sometimes it is written as 'mmol/l' or just 'mM'.

Total cholesterol

The desirable upper limit of total cholesterol (i.e. all the different types put together) is presently considered to be 5 mmol/litre. Total cholesterol is often abbreviated to 'TC'.

LDL

The upper limit of acceptable LDL is 3 mmol/litre.

People with angina who have a total cholesterol level of 5 mmol/litre or more, or LDL of 3 mmol/litre or more, should be offered treatment to reduce their lipid levels.

The methods by which raised cholesterol can be lowered, the importance of cholesterol levels in people who have no evidence of atherosclerosis and the wider implications of taking action on cholesterol are all subjects that are touched upon later in this book.

Electrocardiogram

The electrocardiogram, or ECG, is one of those tests often seen done but which still seems a bit mysterious to the lay person, but the principle behind the ECG is quite straightforward.

All muscles generate a tiny electrical signal when they contract and the ECG machine is basically a very sensitive detector capable of picking up the signals from the heart during each beat. The heart muscle does not all contract at once – what happens is that a wave of electrical activity spreads through the muscle at high speed, starting at a specialised area within the heart that acts as our natural pacemaker. This electrical wave therefore has two qualities that can be measured – direction and speed.

The heart, of course, beats deep within the chest and we can't attach wires to it; however, we don't need to. The human body is made up largely of salty water (admittedly that is a simplification!), and salty water conducts electricity. When someone is connected to an ECG machine a wire is clipped to each wrist and ankle and another wire is connected at a number of positions across the front of the chest (usually using little electrically conducting stickers). From the electrical point of view this is as good as connecting wires around the heart at different places because the arms, legs and chest wall conduct the signals spreading out from the heart very well.

Each of these electrodes is in effect 'looking' at the heart from a different angle. As the electrical wave spreads through the heart muscle then at any one moment the signal picked up by, say, the right arm will be stronger than that at the left ankle, and so on. Of course, this all happens at high speed but by recording the pattern of signals recorded by different combinations of electrodes in a standard way cardiologists have built up a very detailed knowledge of heart muscle behaviour.

One of the many patterns that can often be seen is the effect of a poor blood supply to one area of heart muscle and by examining in which electrode combination this is most obvious a good estimation can often be made of which area of the heart is affected. Other information that can potentially be gained from the ECG includes the electrical rhythm of the heart, evidence of a previous heart attack or of heart muscle thickening (which usually results from untreated high blood pressure).

The great advantage of the ECG is that it is easy, quick and cheap to do. Many general practitioners have their own ECG machine in the surgery, and if not they can easily arrange for the test to be done at the local hospital. Interpreting ECGs is not easy but it is a skill that can be learned and with practice a doctor can read an ECG as easily as a book. The ECG gives a lot of information but it is not a very sensitive test – it can be normal in someone with even severe angina. Nonetheless it gives enough useful information to now be considered an essential test for all people with angina. It also provides a useful record of the heart's activity that can be compared with years later if need be to see if there has been any change.

EXERCISE ECG

The previous section dealt with the 'resting ECG', in which the person having the test lies down and completely relaxes during the process. However, angina is a condition that comes on when a person is doing something active or is under some form of stress. A natural development of the resting ECG was therefore the exercise ECG, in which the same recordings are made but this time while the patient is exercising on a treadmill or bicycle. The benefit of the exercise ECG is that it can reveal areas of heart muscle where the blood supply might be fine at rest, but not under stress. This shows up in the electrical pattern of the ECG and may or may not be accompanied by the symptoms of angina.

The exercise ECG is therefore a very useful tool in diagnosing angina, but its particular advantage is that it can greatly help the heart specialist pick out those people who have more severe coronary heart disease. As we'll see later there are many possible ways to treat angina, some of them involving fairly 'invasive' procedures, and the exercise ECG is commonly used to detect who needs further assessment with this in mind.

Exercise ECG testing is considerably more demanding in equipment, personnel, expertise and back-up than the resting ECG and is only possible in specially equipped units in hospital. It is, however, an extremely helpful test in assessing chest pain. It is not foolproof – 30 per cent of people who have coronary heart disease detected by other methods have a normal exercise ECG – but if someone is able to work to a high level of physical activity during the test without any abnormality in their ECG the degree of CHD they are likely to have (if any) is mild. Exercise tests are particularly helpful, when combined with all the other information known about a person with angina, in deciding if that person is in a low, medium or high risk group for getting further trouble from CHD. This concept of 'risk stratification' is explained more fully in the next chapter.

Not everyone is suitable for exercise ECG testing. Heart-related reasons include some types of ECG abnormality that make it difficult to detect the changes in electrical pattern when the heart's blood supply is poorer, and general medical conditions, such as severe lung disease or arthritis that would stop someone exercising sufficiently hard, would also limit its use.

During the test the person has to work at a sufficient pace to place themselves under enough strain to stress the heart. The technician attending the test, by setting the treadmill to different heights and speeds, can control the amount of effort. These settings are made according to a set of rules, or protocols. The commonest used in the UK is the Bruce protocol. During the test the ECG is taken continuously along with the person's blood pressure and symptoms.

Exercise testing is a safe procedure when done properly and this includes ensuring that people with, for example, very high blood pressure or a degree of heart failure are not put through the test. About once in every 10,000 tests an exercise test can prove too much of a strain and bring on a heart attack or similarly serious problem. This is another reason why exercise testing has to be done in a hospital – so that the full range of medical help is to hand if it is required.

Heart scans

There are two main types of scanning technique that can be used to investigate the blood supply to different parts of the heart and the strength of the heart's pumping action. In addition to providing this information they can also be used to look at people who are unable to undergo exercise ECG testing for any reason.

RADIOACTIVE IMAGING

The medical term for this is 'myocardial perfusion imaging', or MPI (myocardial means anything to do with heart muscle). This test uses a tiny amount of radioactive tracer material, which is injected into the bloodstream of the person having the test. A very sensitive detecting device, called a gamma camera, is able to pick up the radioactivity coming from the tracer material and is positioned over the heart. Over the course of several minutes the gamma camera builds up a picture of which parts of the heart are well supplied with blood and which are poorly supplied, based on the amount of radioactivity displayed by these areas. The tracer's radioactivity fades rapidly, and does no harm to the patient. Tracer materials used are either thallium or technetium.

In order to mimic 'stress' in someone having such a scan it is possible to inject other drugs (dipyridamole or adenosine) which will have the effect of widening the coronary arteries (thus improving the contrast between areas with a good and bad circulation) or by using a drug whose action stimulates the heart to contract (dobutamine).

The images produced by a gamma camera usually use colour to indicate the degree of radioactivity, and hence blood flow. A typical normal image looks like a doughnut, as the heart is visualised in a cross section, as if it had been cut through with a bacon slicer. However, if there is an area of poor circulation this shows up as an area of different colour, as though a bite had been taken out of the doughnut.

Radioactive imaging depends on sophisticated equipment and skilled technicians. It is not available everywhere in the country and is generally only used to assess someone who for one reason or another cannot perform an exercise ECG adequately.

ECHOCARDIOGRAM

The echocardiogram, or 'echo' test, is one that is familiar to most women who have had a baby sometime in the past few decades, and uses the same principles of sound waves and echoes as are used to assess the growing baby inside the womb. High frequency sound is sent through the skin by a probe placed on the skin, and the sound that comes back to the receiver, which is within the same housing, depends on the type of surface that it bounces back from. As the heart is a fluid-filled pump the echo picture can usually distinguish quite well those areas that are muscle and those that are blood. The echo can take repeated pictures very rapidly, so one can see the heart beating very well. Echocardiography, to give it its full title, is very good at investigating murmurs and assessing the thickness and motion of the heart muscle, and it is a routinely used instrument for those sorts of tests. In a few centres some cardiologists also use the echocardiogram as a form of 'stress test'.

Areas of heart muscle that have poorer blood supply do not contract so effectively and this can be detected by the skilled operator. As with radioisotope scans, one can 'stress' the patient using injectable drugs in order to enhance the information obtained from the test. Using the echocardiogram in this way is uncommon – most cardiologists use the information gained from the exercise ECG to assess the patient and the other tests only in particular circumstances.

Angiography

Angiography means outlining the size, shape and connections of blood vessels by injecting a dye into them that shows up on X-rays taken at the same time. To outline the coronary arteries the dye has to be delivered through a narrow flexible tube manoeuvred through the main artery system of the body and then into the coronary circulation.

Clearly this is a much more 'invasive' technique than the preceding tests and requires a high degree of skill on the part of the specialist. The techniques and equipment involved in coronary angiography have, however, now been developed to a very high degree.

Not only does angiography make it possible to see for certain whether there are any significant blockages to the coronary arteries but it also enables the specialist to do something about them. There are several techniques that can be used to open up narrowed arteries using the same methods as angiography, and it is possible both to diagnose CHD and treat it at the same time. These methods are explained in more detail in chapter 7.

When carrying out an angiogram the patient lies on a table within a specially equipped room which also has X-ray equipment capable of taking moving images. A local anaesthetic freezes the skin at the site chosen to access the main artery system of the body, and this is usually at the groin (femoral artery). It is also possible to use the artery at the front of the elbow (brachial artery).

Into this area the doctor inserts a sheath that pierces the artery wall but which has a hollow channel within it through which can be threaded the long flexible catheter tube, itself hollow, used for injecting the dye. This is threaded up first through the main artery of the leg and then through the aorta – the largest of the body's arteries – all the way back to where the aorta starts at its junction with the heart. If you cast your mind back to the earlier description of the coronary circulation you will remember that this is where the two openings lie that lead to the right and the left coronary arteries. The tip of the catheter is specially shaped so that by gentle twisting, pushing and pulling actions it can be guided to the correct place. Snapshots taken by the X-ray machine confirm that the catheter is correctly positioned and then the dye is injected while recording a series of images taken from different directions. An illustration of the results one can get is shown in figure 6.

Chapter 8 covers the process of deciding the best treatment for a person with angina, and where angioplasty fits in to that, but in brief angiography is used when:

- There is disabling angina despite full drug treatment.
- The exercise ECG has suggested 'high risk' coronary artery disease.
- There is uncertainty about whether someone does or does not have angina.

Figure 6: Appearance of the heart arteries in an arteriogram

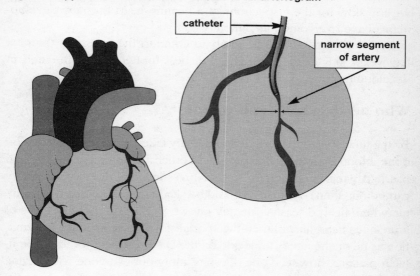

Other techniques

Medical advances continue all the time and there are other methods in development by which images of the heart can be taken. They are not widely available, and their exact role and usefulness are still being investigated, but they have the advantage of not requiring needles, catheters and other forms of invasion of the person having the test.

In magnetic resonance imaging (MRI) scans the patient lies within a magnetic field and then radio pulses are rapidly switched on and off. This causes the water molecules of the body to 'resonate' and in doing so to emit their own radio signal, which the machine detects and translates into an image.

In computerised tomography (CT) scans X-rays are beamed in sequence from all points of a circle around the patient, and a computer then works out the density of the various tissues the beam has passed through, and converts this information to a picture. Older CT scanners are too slow for the fast actions of a beating heart but new developments have overcome this difficulty.

Both MRI and CT will be likely to come to the fore over the next few years, but in the meantime are best thought of as research in development.

Who needs what – and when?

By the time someone has had their history taken, physical examination done, blood pressure, cholesterol and other measurements made, and has had whichever sorts of further investigations that are necessary carried out, then of course it should be clear whether angina is present. Or, where heart disease is already known to exist (perhaps because of a previous heart attack) then the specialist will have as much information as he or she needs to decide on the best treatment for the patient.

In practice, however, one doesn't simply put everyone with angina through the same number of investigations – they are not necessary in everyone and can be potentially harmful in others. Nor is it necessary to wait until the last possible test has been done before making a decision on the diagnosis and a recommendation on treatment.

The purpose of the following chapters is to explain the way in which an individual has his or her particular circumstances assessed and acted upon in a timely and appropriate manner.

Rapid access chest pain clinics

Much of the preceding information has been about high-tech heart investigations but it is worth ending this chapter with a few down-to-earth practical points.

First, it is still too common for people to put up with chest pains for a while before going to the doctor. Even the best equipment is useless if someone with angina keeps it to himself or herself. So if you have started getting chest pains, make that appointment with your doctor now. If you get severe chest pain lasting more than fifteen minutes, call 999.

Second, it defeats the purpose for patients to see their GP and then find themselves waiting several months to see a specialist. Rapid access chest pain clinics should be available in all parts of the country so that people who have recently developed chest pain are quickly assessed by a cardiologist.

Third, it is essential that all patients with angina have their degree of risk assessed with the aims of detecting high risk people as soon as possible as well as offering all patients appropriate advice and treatment. To a large extent that means good access to exercise ECG facilities throughout the UK.

The delivery of such facilities is a core part of the government's commitment to improving coronary heart disease. You should therefore expect to receive this service if your GP thinks you need it – and be willing to ask why if it is still not available in your area.

Chapter 5

Modifying Risk Factors

All human beings are unique, even if nominally suffering from the same medical condition, so two people with angina will have features in common and other features that are different.

The aims of angina assessment are:

- To ensure that the correct diagnosis is made.
- To identify the risk factors for angina and offer advice and treatment for those that can be improved.
- To provide the best treatment for an individual, taking all of their personal factors into account.

Achieving all of this requires a combined approach between the patient, his or her GP (and other primary care professionals) and the heart specialist. This chapter is particularly concerned with what you can do to reduce the chance of CHD developing or getting worse.

Risk assessment

The medical term that takes all of this into account is 'risk assessment'. By this it is meant that every important factor that can influence an individual's risk of developing CHD, or making it worse, is properly addressed. We know that this is not being done consistently well. To take one example, in a recent national population survey only one in eight people who had a history of CHD had a total cholesterol level that was below the target level of 5 mmol/litre. By the end of this chapter you should have a good idea of what risk assessment means in more detail, and can go some way to assessing your own level of risk. Incidentally, cardiologists often use the term 'risk assessment' when referring to the exercise ECG and other such tests that can indicate the severity of a person's coronary disease, but we're using the term here in a more general sense.

Newly diagnosed angina

Earlier in the book we looked at the fact that chest pain can be due to many causes, and that various tests can be done to ensure that the correct diagnosis is made. Where there is a classic history of angina and an expected response to anti-anginal treatment, perhaps with confirmatory findings on the resting ECG that CHD is present, it will be likely that the diagnosis of angina can be made with confidence and acted upon from the start. But the first task, whether or not the diagnosis is obvious, is to assess each of the important risk factors for that individual. (For the sake of simplifying the grammar our 'virtual patient' in the next section is male.)

Risk factor profile

There are seven important questions to be answered:

1 Does he smoke?
2 What is his cholesterol level?

3 What is his blood pressure?
4 Does he have diabetes?
5 What is his weight?
6 Does he have a family history of premature coronary artery disease?
7 What is his age?

We can't choose our parents or make ourselves younger, so questions 6 and 7 help in assessing the likelihood of CHD developing but are not things we can change. (CHD is more common in older people. Being male is also a risk factor for developing CHD.) The first five points are, however, *modifiable* risk factors. (Diabetes can't necessarily be prevented from occurring, but if it is well controlled there is much less chance of developing heart disease.)

Three other important pieces of 'lifestyle' information are needed:

1 What is his diet?
2 How much exercise does he take?
3 How much alcohol does he drink?

These factors have a bearing on several other risks. For example, a high alcohol consumption pushes up blood pressure and contributes to being overweight. Exercise helps reduce weight and improves the proportion of 'good cholesterol' in the blood, and so on. It is important to appreciate that all risk factors are linked in some way or another. As is shown later, risks tend to multiply each other, so some improvement in several risk factors reduces the risk of CHD more effectively than acting on just one or two.

SMOKING
Smoking has a marked effect upon cardiovascular risk and is the single biggest preventable cause of death in the UK. Stopping smoking is the top priority for any individual, and especially so for people with angina and/or a past history of heart attack. People with angina who continue to smoke are five times more likely to have a heart attack over the

ensuing ten years compared to angina sufferers who stop smoking. Several other studies show convincingly that, for someone who has a heart attack, the risk of having another one over the next five years is approximately halved by stopping smoking.

The extent of the heart risk increases with the number of cigarettes smoked, but there is no 'safe' number to smoke. Put another way, the only 'safe' number to smoke is zero. When someone stops smoking, their heart risk begins to fall but it is uncertain how long it takes to fall to that of someone who has never smoked. It is generally thought that two to three years after stopping smoking the risk of developing CHD is halved and by ten years it is about the same as for a non-smoker. If that puts you off even trying because you think it will take too long to see any benefit, the good news is that a large part of the improvement occurs within the first year or so, and then it begins to tail off. It is therefore never too late to stop smoking. Remember too that we are not talking here about the risk of developing lung cancer or any of the other smoking-related diseases, all of which you will make less likely by giving up the habit.

Getting help to stop smoking is easier than it used to be. Nicotine replacement doubles a person's chance of quitting and medication such as amfebutamone (bupropion, Zyban) is also effective. Both these types of medication are prescribable by GPs who can also, as with all of the risk factors covered in this book, offer additional help, support and advice. Nicotine replacement can also be bought from the pharmacist without a prescription. On-line support and information on stopping smoking is available free on NetDoctor at http://community.netdoktor.com/ccs/uk/smoking/index.jsp and other sources of information are listed in appendix C.

CHOLESTEROL

It is a good idea for all adults to have their cholesterol checked, and preferably to do so long before any health problems related to high cholesterol reveal themselves. It is essential for people who have CHD to have their total cholesterol (TC) brought as much as possible to within the target area of below 5 mmol/litre. The low density lipo-protein (LDL) level should also be below 3 mmol/litre and if either condition is not met then that person needs cholesterol lowering advice and treatment. Controlling blood lipids to within these limits helps to stop plaque building up within the coronary arteries and can even reduce the size of plaque already there.

In someone with angina who also has a high blood cholesterol level it is probably better to simultaneously start on a cholesterol-lowering diet and medication rather than trying a diet first and then adding cholesterol-lowering treatment only when the diet alone has failed. Waiting for the diet to work, and only treating those people whose cholesterol does not fall far enough, exposes the person to higher levels of cholesterol for longer and results in a greater likelihood of developing more severe CHD. Recent research also shows that when you compare two groups of people with the same blood cholesterol level, but in whom one group is taking 'statin' drugs (see chapter 6) to achieve that cholesterol level, the statin group have fewer coronary events than the other group. This suggests an extra benefit from statin drugs beyond their cholesterol-lowering effect, and this is currently the focus of much medical interest and research.

When the total cholesterol is raised to 8mmol/litre or above there is a high chance that this is due to an inherited condition and so other family members need also to have their cholesterol level checked. People with such high levels of cholesterol should also be seen by a specialist in lipid abnormalities.

DIET, FAT AND CHD

Some fat is essential in our diet. Fats provide a source of concentrated energy and contain the essential fat-soluble vitamins A, D, E and K. The two main types of dietary fat are 'saturated' and 'unsaturated'. Saturated fats are solid at room temperature and are more undesirable from the health point of view. They are found mainly in lard, red meat, suet, dripping, eggs and full-fat dairy products. They are also found in hard margarines – which are often used for making cakes, biscuits and pastry. Unsaturated fats are generally liquid at room temperature and come from vegetable sources but are also found in oily fish and in soft margarines labelled 'high in polyunsaturates'. These unsaturated fats contain essential fatty acids that cannot be manufactured by the body and need to be obtained from food. 'Omega-3' and 'omega-6' fatty acids are types found in oily fish and they appear to give additional protection against cardiovascular disease.

When people in specialised hospital units keep stringently to diets low in cholesterol and saturated fats they can lower their cholesterol by 10–15 per cent but in the setting of the community only 3–5 per cent lowering of cholesterol is found by diet alone, mainly because people find it difficult to stick to the diets long term. Although the amount of change in cholesterol brought about by diet is modest it is still worthwhile, as for every 1 per cent fall in cholesterol there is a 2–3 per cent drop in likelihood of CHD. Taking a broader view of fat in the diet is more rewarding as studies on heart attack survivors who increased the amount of fish in their diet showed they were significantly less likely to have a further and fatal heart attack within the following two years.

Another study, in which a similar group of patients was put on a 'Mediterranean style' diet (more bread, vegetables, cereals, fruit and fish and less meat and dairy produce), was stopped early because the people on the Mediterranean diet were doing substantially better than the comparison group on their ordinary diet. This reveals one of the most important points about any risk factor and CHD, which is that lifestyle changes can have as much or more of an effect than any medication.

In summary, the diet changes that benefit heart disease risk are:

- Increased fruit and vegetable consumption to five portions per day.
- Increased oil-rich fish consumption to three portions per week.
- Decreased total fat consumption, increasing the proportion of unsaturated fat.
- Increased amount of starchy food and reduced amount of sugary food in the diet.

Appendix D contains a checklist for you to assess your present diet and see where you might need to make changes.

BLOOD PRESSURE

Raised blood pressure increases the strain on arteries and the heart and is one of the most important factors to raise the risk of developing atherosclerosis. If angina is present then the importance of getting the blood pressure down to acceptable levels is much increased.

High blood pressure is covered fully in a companion book in this series, so only the most important facts are presented here.

Each beat of the heart sends a pulse of pressure through all of the arteries of the body, propelling blood around the circulation. The maximum pressure developed during this action is called the 'systolic pressure'. Blood pressure falls while the heart is refilling in readiness for the next beat, but not to zero – the stretchiness of our arteries goes on squeezing the blood vessel system – and the minimum pressure reached at this part of the cycle is the 'diastolic pressure'. Blood pressure is always measured in millimetres of mercury (written as mmHg), which comes from the fact that blood pressure measuring devices use the height of a column of mercury as the standard against which to gauge the pressure.

In angina the top level of acceptable systolic pressure is 140 mmHg and of diastolic pressure it is 85 mmHg. The shorthand way of writing this is 140/85. If either of the systolic or diastolic readings is consistently above these levels then treatment to lower the blood pressure to within target levels is required. This might mean simple dietary salt restriction and weight loss if the rise is small, or long-term blood pressure lowering medication if simple measures fail.

If you do have raised blood pressure the most useful things you can do to help yourself are:

- ***Reduce the amount of salt in your diet.***
  Ideally you should take less than 5 grams of salt daily, which is enough to fill a teaspoon. But remember that this has to include all

of the salt that comes in processed foods and in practice could mean you are presently taking three to five times the amount of salt you actually need.

- *Increase the amount of fresh fruit and vegetables in your diet.*
  These contain potassium, which is also a salt but, unlike sodium, which is in common table salt and bad for blood pressure, increased potassium in the diet helps lower blood pressure.

- *Take more exercise.*
  You don't need to become an athlete to get the benefits. A brisk walk three times a week lasting about 20-40 minutes will lower blood pressure, and ideally you should aim to exercise every day. (For people with angina who are starting an exercise regime or whose symptoms presently limit their capacity for exercise, please check with your doctor or nurse for advice on how to build up your exercise level safely.)

- *Keep alcohol consumption to about 1 or 2 units daily.*
  Consuming a small amount of alcohol daily (up to two standard units) appears to have a beneficial effect upon cardiovascular risk. There are many possible explanations for this, but among the most likely are that compounds within some alcoholic drinks, particularly red wine, mop up 'free radical' molecules that are capable of causing tissue damage. However, the effects rapidly turn from beneficial to harmful when higher levels of alcohol are consumed. The usual recommended maximum consumption of alcohol per week is 21 units for women and 28 units of alcohol for men, but people with angina should limit their drinking to 14 units per week for women and 21 units per week for men (SIGN guidelines). A unit of alcohol is:

  a) 250ml (1/2 pint) of ordinary strength beer / lager
  b) 1 glass (125ml / 4 fl oz) of wine
  c) 1 pub measure of sherry / vermouth (1.5oz.)
  d) 1 pub measure of spirits (1.5oz.)

- *Keep your body weight to the ideal range.*

BODY WEIGHT

Excess body weight has several adverse effects upon cardiovascular disease. It increases blood pressure, cholesterol and triglyceride levels, makes it more likely that someone will develop diabetes (see below) and puts an increased strain on the heart, increasing its requirement for oxygen and hence blood supply.

Weight and height are related and knowledge of both is needed before one can say if a person is overweight. A simple mathematical formula relating the two is now universally used to do this – the Body Mass Index (BMI). To calculate a BMI, take the person's weight (in kilograms) and divide it by the square of their height (in metres). For example, an 80kg person of height 1.7m will have a BMI of $80/(1.7 \times 1.7) = 27.7$ kg/m^2 (the BMI formula applies equally to men and women). The ranges of BMI are:

- Normal   = 20–24.9
- Overweight = 25–30
- Obese   = Over 30

The target for anyone with angina is to get their BMI under 25. Table 1 shows a range of heights and the associated weights for the normal and obese ranges.

Losing weight

The healthiest way to lose weight is a sensible combination of diet and exercise. Exercise needs to be started at a low level – short walks, for example, if you are out of condition, with the walks then increased slowly. Introduce dietary changes gradually too – you are trying to alter your behaviour in a way you can keep going with, perhaps forever. Crash diets don't work – they usually end up with you feeling weaker or giving up completely in desperation. This in turn can lead to a yo-yoing effect of weight loss/weight gain.

Eating 300 to 500 calories less per day may lead to losing between one and two pounds (0.5–1 kg) per week. This is a realistic rate of

Table 1: Body mass index guide

Height (less shoes)			Weight range (kg)	Obese weight (kg)
Metres	Feet	Inches	for BMI 20–24.9	for BMI >30
1.50	4	11	45–56	68
1.52	5	0	46–58	69
1.54	5	1	47–59	71
1.56	5	1	49–61	73
1.58	5	2	50-62	75
1.60	5	3	51–64	77
1.62	5	4	52–66	79
1.64	5	5	53–67	81
1.66	5	5	55–69	83
1.68	5	6	56–71	85
1.70	5	7	58-72	87
1.72	5	8	59-74	89
1.74	5	8	61-75	91
1.76	5	9	62-77	93
1.78	5	10	63-79	95
1.80	5	11	65-81	97
1.82	6	0	66-83	99
1.84	6	0	68-85	102
1.86	6	1	69-86	104
1.88	6	2	71-88	106
1.90	6	3	72-90	108

weight loss. It may seem slow, but if sustained would add up to more than 4 stones (26 kg) in a year. Having a glass of water instead of juice, eating less lunch than usual and having smaller portions of the food you enjoy are all ways to reduce calorie intake without having to necessarily alter your diet significantly. Avoid a second helping at dinner and snacks between meals, which may have become a habit.

Cut down on beer and alcohol. All these things will influence your health in a positive way.

DIABETES

Diabetes increases the risk for CHD up to fourfold. There are two main types of diabetes – Type 1 is that found in younger people (under 35 approximately) and is due to insufficient or absent production of the hormone insulin by the pancreas gland inside the abdomen. Insulin is necessary to control the body's use of glucose – the main energy source for our tissues – and Type 1 diabetes always needs to be treated with insulin injections.

Type 2 diabetes is much more common (over 90 per cent of diabetes) and occurs in people of middle age or older. They tend to be overweight and essentially do not produce enough insulin for their needs. As many as half of the people who have Type 2 diabetes are unaware of it – their symptoms may be so mild they do not seek medical advice for them until years later. (Type 1 diabetes always causes enough symptoms to get noticed.)

Type 2 diabetes can be treated by diet alone, or by diet plus tablets to lower the blood sugar. In both types of diabetes the typical symptoms include thirst, frequent passage of urine, tiredness, tendency to thrush infection and weight loss. In diabetes all cardiovascular risk factors are magnified in effect, so particular efforts need to be made to reduce excess weight, lower blood cholesterol if it is high and to take more exercise – a high proportion of people with Type 2 diabetes are both overweight and sedentary.

Further details on diabetes management are outside the scope of this book but are covered in a companion volume in the series. There is good evidence to show that people with poorly controlled diabetes are at greater risk of medical complications than those whose blood sugar control is tight. The presence of angina implies that a degree of CHD is already present, which increases the importance of good diabetic management.

Multiple risks, multiple effects

When we look at the combined effects of multiple risk factors we can see clearly how important it is to take the whole person into consideration, rather than a single measurement. Look at figure 7, which illustrates the interplay of three main risk factors that we can modify (as opposed to those that we cannot modify, such as our sex or race).

Figure 7: Interaction of the main risk factors for heart disease

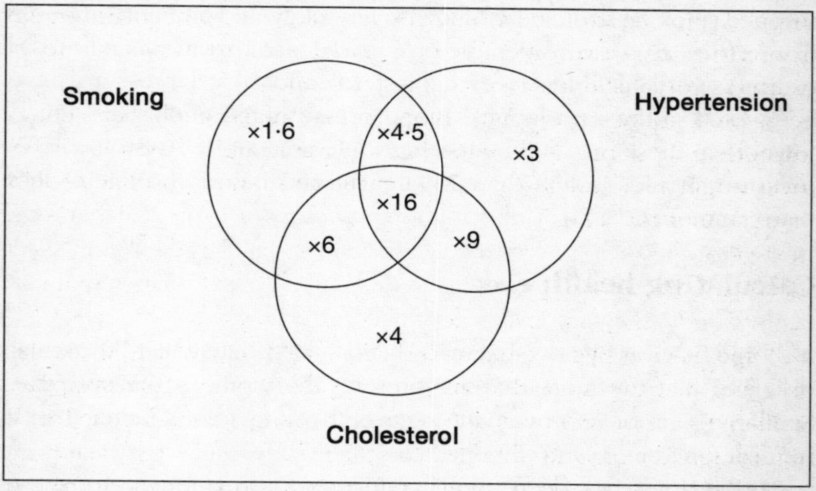

In the figure there are three circles – one each for hypertension, smoking and raised cholesterol – and you will see that they all overlap. The numbers within each main area represent the increase in risk of developing coronary heart disease that would be experienced by a middle-aged non-smoker with normal blood pressure and blood cholesterol were he to have any of these three risk factors:

1 Systolic blood pressure of 195 mmHg
2 Blood cholesterol raised to 8.25 mmol/l or more
3 Smoking to any extent

For example, if this person took up smoking he would increase his chance of getting coronary heart disease by 1.6 times. If his cholesterol went up to 8.25 mmol/l his risk would increase by 4 times. If he had both raised cholesterol and smoked the risk would be 6 times greater – the overlap between the two areas. In the middle is someone with all three risk factors, whose risk is 16 times greater than the low-risk individual. This diagram makes it clear not only that multiple risk factors greatly increase the likelihood of CHD, but also that removing a modifiable risk factor is very beneficial. If our 'man in the middle' stopped smoking and did nothing else his risk would in theory improve from x16 to x9 – a considerable drop. Note also that in this particular example very high levels of cholesterol and blood pressure have been used in the calculations. Blood pressure and cholesterol levels lower than these may still be too high. (Remember that systolic blood pressure should be less than 140 mmHg and blood cholesterol less than 5 mmol/l.)

Calculating health risk

It should be clear by now that many factors contribute to cardiovascular risk, and that the more that are present, the worse is the outcome. Similarly, a bit of improvement in several risk factors is better than a lot of improvement in only one.

This chapter has been about collecting information in someone with angina – although it might as well have been for any number of other medical reasons. This is basic health information and ought to be known for everyone, yet only a minority of people with known CHD have all of this information recorded in their medical file. Consequently an accurate estimation of coronary risk is impossible, or at best is likely to be inaccurate, in many people for whom the information is of crucial importance. As we will see later, many decisions on the treatment of CHD are currently being made within the NHS on cost grounds, but are being justified on the basis of treating the most 'at risk' people first. Given that the information base for these decisions is very inadequate, such decisions need to be called in to question.

In chapter 10 we take an overview of the practicalities of dealing with CHD risk in the population, but most people reading this book are likely to already have angina. As such they deserve that treatment decisions are based upon the best possible information, and that means that all relevant information about them has been gathered and properly assessed.

Such are the pressures on the NHS and such is the evidence from the medical literature, that it is not safe to assume that all risk factors have been properly addressed in every individual.

From your own point of view, if you have angina you should ensure that you have been assessed in each of the risk factor areas that have been outlined in this chapter. You should know your blood pressure, cholesterol, blood glucose, BMI, etc. Knowing this, along with your medical history, allows a proper assessment of your 'risk profile', and consequently the best line of treatment for you if you have angina.

There are now well worked out guidelines to advise doctors how to best treat someone with angina and the purpose of chapter 8 is to take you through that process. Before doing so you need to know the basics of the drugs and other treatments available for treating angina.

Chapter 6

Drug Treatments for Angina

As we've seen, angina largely results from the narrowing of the heart's arteries from the process called atherosclerosis. As a result there is inadequate delivery of blood to the heart when it is under increased load. Treatments for angina have therefore developed along the following lines:

1 Those that increase blood flow to the heart.
2 Those that decrease the workload of the heart.

In addition to these are:

3 The treatments which slow down the process of atherosclerosis.

To some extent these divisions are artificial – several drugs, for example, work both to increase the heart's blood flow *and* to reduce the workload on heart muscle, but it is a good enough classification to hold in our mind when we look at how the drugs are used in practice.

In achieving all of these aims both medical (i.e. drug) and physical (i.e. surgical) treatments have evolved. This chapter covers drug treatments, and chapter 7 looks at surgical or 'intervention' treatments.

Classes of drug treatments

There are four main types, or class, of anti-anginal drug:

1 Beta blockers
2 Calcium channel blockers
3 Potassium channel activator (presently only one available)
4 Nitrates

BETA BLOCKERS

The way in which our nervous system sends signals from nerve to nerve and from nerve to tissue is complex but essentially is a combination of electrical impulses and of 'chemical messengers'. These messenger molecules are often the final step in the signalling process and the release of minute amounts at a nerve ending will be what triggers a response from, for example, the tissue to which the nerve is connected.

The adrenal glands are two walnut-sized pieces of highly specialised tissue that sit one above each kidney. They are part of both the nervous system (to which they are connected by many nerve fibres) and of the hormone-producing glands of the body. It was shown in the late nineteenth century that material extracted from the adrenal glands would cause a rise in blood pressure if injected into an animal, and soon afterwards adrenaline was identified as the active substance.

There are several adrenaline-like substances that are manufactured and used within the body as the chemical messengers of the nervous system – noradrenaline is the other main one. Work done in the 1940s showed that these compounds acted upon two types of receptor molecules, named alpha and beta, which were present in different tissues and allowed adrenaline and noradrenaline to have different effects, depending on which receptors they met. Research then showed that there were actually subgroups of both types of receptor. Beta-1 receptors in the heart respond to adrenaline by increasing the heart rate and the force of contraction, and beta-2 receptors in the airway tubes of the lung respond by opening the tubes wider.

Action of beta blockers

Sir James Black won the Nobel Prize in 1988 for his work at ICI in the 1950s and 60s, which led to the invention of propranolol – the first beta blocker drug. Beta blockers reduce the workload of the heart by causing a fall in blood pressure and by reducing the overall force of the heart's pumping action. Beta blockers have been shown to improve the survival rate of people following a heart attack and are a mainstay of treatment in that situation, and for angina in general.

An undesirable effect of beta blockers is that they can narrow the airways of the lungs. This is really only seen in people who also have asthma, but it usually means that the drugs cannot be used in an asthmatic person.

There are about a dozen beta blockers licensed for use in angina and although there may not be much difference between them in efficacy the commonest used are atenolol, bisoprolol and metoprolol.

Side effects caused by beta blockers generally include: tiredness, slow pulse, cold hands and feet, worsening of wheeze, sleep disturbance and digestive system upset.

CALCIUM CHANNEL BLOCKERS

Each individual cell of the body needs to maintain its own internal chemical environment so that the processes of life, such as energy use, cell repair and division and the specific functions of tissue cells, can be carried out. The membrane of a cell is its surrounding wall and far from being an inert container to keep the cell contents tidy the cell membrane is intensely active and carries out numerous chemical processes.

Action of calcium channel blockers

Within cells the concentration of electrically charged atoms (ions) is of great importance to their function. In muscle cells, such as those that surround arteries and arterioles and which therefore determine the size of those blood vessels, the concentration of calcium ions within the muscle cell is kept lower than the fluid outside the cell by 'pumps' within the cell membrane. When a muscle cell is triggered to contract the process involves the opening of calcium channels within the membrane – atomic gates we could say – that allow calcium to flood into the cell, thus stimulating it to contract. Once the contraction phase is over the cell is restored to the relaxed state by the calcium pumps, which transport the excess calcium within the cell back to the outside. By blocking the calcium channels using specially designed drugs the arterioles can be stopped from contracting, which lowers blood pressure.

Calcium channel blockers (some people use the term 'calcium antagonists' instead) are therefore widely used in treating high blood pressure, but their action also takes the load off the heart, and so they are very useful anti-anginal drugs too. They also have direct effects upon the heart muscle cells and upon the tissues within the heart that conduct electrical impulses from the pacemaker tissue. As a result, the calcium channel blockers are not all the same when it comes to their individual effects upon the heart, and this has a significant effect upon the choice of these drugs in angina.

On the basis of their detailed chemical structure there are three types of calcium channel blocker:

1 Nifedipine, amlodipine (and others like them, collectively called dihydropyridines)
2 Verapamil
3 Diltiazem

Verapamil tends to reduce the pumping ability and to slow the electrical activity of the heart. It cannot therefore be used in heart failure, and in particular should not be combined with a beta blocker drug as this could reduce heart output severely. (This is important because it can often be necessary in angina to combine drugs in order to adequately relieve symptoms.)

Diltiazem has some of these problems but can be combined with caution with a beta blocker. This braking effect on the heart shown by verapamil and diltiazem has led to them commonly being called 'rate limiting' calcium channel blockers. As we shall see later this makes them useful if a person with angina cannot take a beta blocker (e.g. because of asthma). The commonest side effects of verapamil are constipation, flushing, headaches, stomach upsets, fatigue and swelling of the ankles. Diltiazem is similar but less likely to cause constipation.

Amlodipine is the most commonly used calcium channel blocker and is described in Appendix B.

Other calcium channel blockers in regular use include felodipine, nifedipine, nicardipine and nisoldipine. All of the preceding calcium channel blockers may be used for angina. Others presently licensed only for high blood pressure are isradipine, lacidipine and lercanidipine.

POTASSIUM CHANNEL ACTIVATOR

There is presently only one drug in this group – nicorandil. As with calcium, potassium has its own role in the life of the cell and nicorandil's effect on smooth muscle cells makes them relax, thus widening blood vessels. It has some actions in common with nitrates too, as it also releases nitric oxide and thereby dilates blood vessels by a different mechanism of action.

Like other drugs that cause dilation of vessels the usual side effects are flushing, headaches and dizziness. Until recently nicorandil tended to be used as an 'add-on' treatment when someone's angina proved difficult to control despite full dosages of the other anti-anginal drugs. However, very recent research data shows that nicorandil has a protective role in CHD. It is therefore likely that it is set to be used far more often than at present.

NITRATES

The ability of chemicals called nitrates to alleviate angina was discovered in the mid-nineteenth century. At that time amyl nitrite was first tried, and subsequently glyceryl trinitrate was used. Glyceryl trinitrate is chemically the same as nitroglycerine, from which dynamite is made, but has no explosive qualities in the form used in medicine!

Action of nitrates

Nitrates work by relaxing 'smooth muscle' – which is the type of muscle that lines veins, arteries and arterioles (small arteries). They do so by releasing nitric oxide – which was mentioned in chapter 2 in connection with its apparent role in the development of atherosclerosis. When this type of smooth muscle relaxes, the blood vessels widen (dilate). Nitrates work both by increasing the flow of blood to an area of heart muscle with a poor blood supply and by reducing the workload on the heart and they do so in several ways.

First, the general widening of the veins throughout the body increases the capacity of this part of the circulation, which therefore acts better as a sort of reservoir for blood. In turn this reduces the rate at which blood flows back to the heart, which reduces the filling pressure of blood within the heart. This pressure partially determines the rate at which the heart has to work, so by lowering it the heart's need for oxygen is reduced.

This drop in heart output, added to by the widening of the general artery system, causes the person's blood pressure to fall, which further takes the load off the heart. This fall in blood pressure can cause symptoms if it is too marked – it can lead to someone feeling dizzy on standing, for example, but in practice people get used to the effect and it tends not to be a major problem.

Within the heart's blood vessels the action is slightly different and to explain it requires a bit more information about the heart's arteries.

We have already seen that there are three main arteries supplying blood to particular territories of heart muscle but when one looks in more detail one sees that there are thousands of tiny connecting arteries which join each main artery's 'territory' with its neighbours. As an analogy, think of a motorway travelling through a city: most of the traffic travels on the motorway, but there is also a surrounding network of minor roads that connect with it and with each other; if an obstruction develops in one part of the system then cars can take a few detours and get round the hold-up. In the body the medical term for this mesh of interconnecting blood vessels is the 'collateral' system. The heart is particularly well supplied with collaterals, which is probably the way that it has evolved precisely to ensure the maximum efficiency of its blood supply. The extent of development of the collaterals can much reduce the impact of a major blockage.

The effect of nitrate drugs within the heart is particularly to dilate the collateral vessels, thus improving the flow of blood to the area in short supply. Doing so does of course 'steal' some blood from the other parts of the heart that are served by normal-sized arteries, but those areas are connected to other areas by collaterals too, so the distribution of blood within the heart muscle evens out.

Forms of nitrates

The most traditional way to use nitrates is in the form of tablets of glyceryl trinitrate placed under the tongue (or inside the cheek). Saliva within the mouth dissolves the tablet, which is immediately absorbed directly by the circulation of blood in the mouth lining. Within just a few seconds of popping the tablet in the mouth the nitrate is flowing through the bloodstream and can be acting to relieve angina. This rapid action is one of the most useful aspects of nitrate drugs and, in addition to their powerful ability to relieve angina, maintains their position among the most popular of treatments.

Nitrates act upon the whole of the circulatory system, not just the blood vessels of the heart, and their main side effects relate largely to this fact. One can therefore get an unpleasant throbbing headache shortly after using a glyceryl trinitrate (GTN) tablet, because of dilation of the blood vessels within the head, or become flushed for the same reason. As mentioned, dizziness can be a problem, especially on standing up too quickly – a good tip when using GTN is to sit down first – and some people experience a racing pulse. Some people are particularly sensitive to the effects of nitrates and need to be careful with the dose that they take. (More details on all of the drugs used in angina are in appendix B.)

A practical problem with GTN tablets is that the active ingredient readily evaporates, so they eventually lose their effect. They should therefore be kept tightly closed in their storage bottle until needed and tablets older than eight weeks should be replaced. GTN sprays are miniature pressurised canisters containing the drug, one spray under the tongue being the equivalent of a tablet, but because the canisters are sealed the spray lasts very much longer and is therefore more practical in use, especially for someone who needs GTN only occasionally.

There are dozens of proprietary types of nitrate in use but they fall into three groups:

1 *Quick-acting tablets and sprays.*
These mostly use glyceryl trinitrate, but another drug, isosorbide dinitrate, can be used in this way too. Although GTN acts quickly its effect wears off after 20–30 minutes. Isosorbide dinitrate has a slower onset of action, but lasts longer.
2 *Longer-acting tablets and capsules.*
These are designed to work over several hours and come in various forms. Some are effective when given just once daily, others need to be used two (rarely three) times a day. Glyceryl trinitrate and isosorbide dinitrate can be used this way as can the third commonly used nitrate – isosorbide mononitrate.
3 *Patches.*
The patches are self-adhesive and look a bit like sticking plasters. They all use glyceryl trinitrate held within a slow-release form that is gradually absorbed through the skin. They need to be changed every day and the idea is that they provide the wearer with a

continuous, low-level amount of nitrate. Although some people do get on quite well with patches they are no better at relieving angina than the oral preparations, and some people find that their skin reacts against the adhesive.

Nitrate tolerance

Before leaving nitrates, one other practical point needs mentioning. It seems that many people who use long-acting nitrates (tablets, capsules or patches) become tolerant of the drug, which results in it losing effectiveness. To get round this it is necessary for the amount of nitrate in the person's body to be reduced to a low level for 4–8 hours during every 24 hours. The best time for this to happen is of course when the heart has least work to do – during sleep. This can conveniently be done by:

- Removing the patch (if used) at bedtime.
- Taking the last dose of a twice-daily preparation no later than about 2 p.m.
- Taking a once-daily preparation in the morning.

This trick appears to prevent nitrate tolerance from happening, and keeps the drug effective every day.

OTHER DRUGS USED IN ANGINA – 'SECONDARY PREVENTION'

The preceding part of this chapter dealt with those drugs that specific-ally act upon angina symptoms. The two other main types of drug that will be commonly used in someone with angina are intended to reduce the further development of blockage within arteries – a process also known as 'secondary prevention'.

Aspirin

Aspirin, properly called acetylsalicylic acid, was first produced in the late nineteenth century and has been one of the most important drugs ever invented. Natural sources of the simpler compound, salicylic acid, such as willow bark and oil of wintergreen, have long been known for their ability to relieve rheumatism, and for most of the first century of aspirin's use it was the benchmark anti-inflammatory painkiller. The more recent discovery of aspirin's effect on blood clotting opened a completely new field of use for the drug.

Circulating within our blood are large numbers of tiny particles called platelets. These are much smaller than the red cells that carry oxygen or the white cells of the immune system, and their main role is to help blood to clot when needed. Normally platelets stay separate but they will clump together under the influence of chemical changes that occur at the site of a cut, for example. When the lining cells (endothelium) of blood vessels are damaged they release trigger substances that cause platelets to stick together at the site of injury. These trigger substances also activate the complex series of reactions within blood that cause it to clot. Platelets, red blood cells and a protein called fibrin, formed by the clotting mechanism, all gather together into a very effective localised blood clot (thrombus) that plugs the breach.

Aspirin reduces the tendency of platelets to stick together and so makes the formation of clots much less likely. In the doses used for this purpose it has only a minimal effect on the time a cut takes to stop bleeding.

When the lining covering a plaque breaks down (the causes of this breakdown are not yet understood) then the underlying fatty deposit and muscle layer is exposed, triggering the local formation of a clot. In a heart attack a coronary artery narrowed by a plaque but which is otherwise stable suddenly becomes unstable and can become totally blocked by the new clot. Aspirin much reduces the chance of this happening. It is therefore now standard practice to give aspirin to everyone with angina or a history of heart attack. Not everyone can take aspirin – for example in some people it can cause indigestion or even a stomach ulcer, and for those people an alternative 'anti-platelet' drug should be used. Clopidogrel (Plavix) is likely to become the most commonly used aspirin alternative although there are others.

Statins

Drugs to lower cholesterol can act in one of several possible ways – by reducing the manufacture of cholesterol by the liver, by binding to cholesterol within the digestive system (preventing its re-absorption back into the bloodstream) or by other actions on the way lipoproteins are handled by the body. Statins act by reducing cholesterol synthesis and are now the major drugs used in cholesterol control. Drugs acting in the other ways are still in use but are more within the realm of the specialist in lipids and are not covered further here.

Statins work by reducing the activity of a key enzyme (called HMG-CoA reductase) used by cells in cholesterol synthesis. Most, although not all, cells that synthesise cholesterol are within the liver. Reduction of cholesterol output is accompanied by a greater uptake of low density lipoprotein (LDL) by liver cells, thereby lowering the amount of LDL in the blood. LDL, as you will remember from chapter 4, is 'bad cholesterol', and lowering LDL lowers a person's chance of getting CHD.

Statins are well-tolerated drugs with relatively few side effects. Minor reactions include indigestion and diarrhoea. More significant, but rarer, reactions include allergic rashes and abnormalities in liver tests. Even rarer is a type of muscle inflammation called myositis. Myositis should be suspected if someone on a statin develops muscle pains and it can be further investigated by blood tests. Similarly, a watch every few months on the liver can be carried out by blood tests, although mild abnormalities do not necessarily mean that the drug has to be stopped. Using a statin therefore carries with it a need for monitoring, but this can be kept to a reasonable level. There are presently four statins in use: atorvastatin, fluvastatin, pravastatin and simvastatin. The main research data showing the benefits of statins was conducted on pravastatin and simvastatin (see appendix A for references). Simvastatin is described in more detail in appendix B.

An area of great interest at the moment concerns the overall effect of statins on the risk of CHD, as their benefit appears to extend beyond the fact that they effectively lower cholesterol in the blood. Improvements in CHD risk have been seen with statins irrespective of the 'starting' level of cholesterol within the range 4–8 mmol/litre, which of course includes levels of cholesterol that we would currently consider to be 'normal'. It seems that statins may have a direct effect on the plaque within diseased arteries, making them less liable to break down with the sudden clotting just described.

This does not necessarily mean that vast numbers of apparently healthy people ought to be taking statins – coronary risk has many aspects and smokers will still need to stop smoking, for example – but it does mean that the exact role of statins and the consequent cost considerations of using them are one of the most important topics under consideration in CHD. More on this subject is presented in chapter 10.

Chapter 7

'Intervention' Treatments for Angina

The term 'intervention' is used here to refer to all of the treatments presently available for angina in which some form of physical or surgical method is used. At one end of the scale is conventional surgery in which someone has an operation under general anaesthetic to bypass blocked coronary arteries, but in the field of heart disease there has been a huge increase in recent years of treatments that can be conducted on the heart and coronary arteries while the patient remains fully alert and is subjected to minimal invasion.

Balloons and stents

We touched on these methods in chapter 4 when discussing angiograms – the X-ray outlines of the coronary arteries that can be obtained by injecting dye through a long thin catheter tube guided through the artery system of the body. Virtually the same techniques can be used to introduce miniature instruments that can be delivered to the narrowed coronary artery and then used to widen the tight segment.

TERMS IN USE

Some jargon terms often crop up in this area and are best explained now:

- *Revascularisation*: any technique intended to improve blood flow to an area whose blood supply is blocked. Usually limited to the intervention methods (as opposed to drugs that can dissolve clots, for example).
- *Percutaneous*: literally 'through the skin'. Used when talking about interventions that can be done under local anaesthetic by inserting instruments through the skin to reach an artery and then manipulating them into position within the heart.
- *Transluminal*: means 'going through the inside of a tube'.
- *-plasty*: added to the end of a word when referring to any sort of operation.

So the term 'percutaneous coronary interventions' or 'PCI' just means any of those techniques in which the specialist introduces some sort of device that is then manipulated into the coronary arteries.

PTCA

The commonest technique is called 'percutaneous transluminal coronary angioplasty', or PTCA for short. Figure 8 illustrates the principle behind the technique.

As with the angiogram, the doctor freezes the skin over the artery chosen for access – which is usually the femoral artery as it is easily located at the front of the groin. Under X-ray guidance a fine-bore tube is passed up the aorta until it reaches the right or left coronary artery. The special shape of the catheter allows it to be manipulated into the best position. Once correctly placed the doctor can then pass

Figure 8: PTCA explained

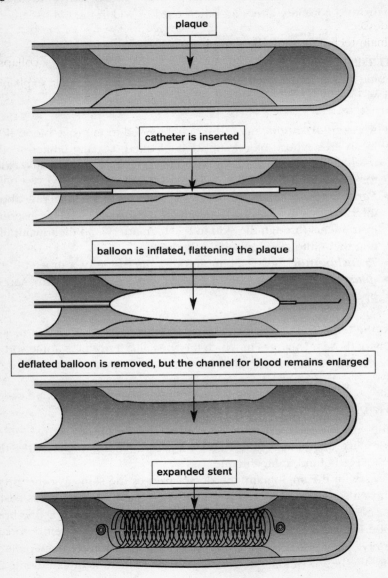

a very fine guide wire through the tube and on through the partially obstructed coronary artery. When the guide wire is in place other devices can be slid over it in order to carry out the procedure. Two main techniques are then employed.

First one can use a miniature balloon, introduced in a collapsed state until it lies within the narrowed part of the coronary artery, and attached by its own tube back to a syringe held by the doctor. Once correctly positioned the doctor can apply pressure to the syringe, which inflates the balloon and flattens the plaque, creating a wider channel than before.

In the original technique the balloon and other tubes and wires would then be withdrawn and the procedure was over. As you might imagine there was a subsequent tendency for the flattened plaque to swell up again and so the problem would slowly recur. The technique has therefore been improved by introducing a metal 'stent' or wire cage at the site of the plaque in order to keep the area open. The stent is wrapped around the balloon and the whole assembly is introduced in its collapsed state, as described above, until it is in the correct position. When the balloon is inflated so too is the metal stent, but the stent keeps its shape thereafter, so reducing the chance of the artery closing up again (see the last part of figure 8).

RISKS AND BENEFITS OF PTCA

PTCA and 'stenting' are obviously techniques that require great skill, but they have made a significant difference to the ability of cardiologists to treat people with severely narrowed coronary arteries and are much less 'invasive' than major surgery. They can therefore be used on a wider range of people, including those who would be unable to withstand the greater demands on the body of a major operation.

As with any operation, however, there is some attached risk. Possible complications include bleeding from the coronary artery, or blockage and a subsequent heart attack. In the worst case death can result. In practice such outcomes are rare – estimates of the average risk of dying from PTCA are less than 0.5 per cent of the procedures.

The main problem with PTCA is re-closure of the narrowed area, which used to occur in up to 30 per cent of people who have it done. The medical term for this is 're-stenosis'. Improvement in techniques (particularly stenting) has lowered this rate to about 10 per cent and further improvements are seen by using routine anti-platelet medication at the time of placing the stent.

The main benefit of PTCA compared with drug treatment alone is improvement of angina symptoms. In selected patients this improvement is usually substantial but the exact level of improvement can vary a lot from person to person.

As with any complex treatment, it is necessary for each person to be assessed on their own merits. If resources and facilities within the UK were evenly distributed then one could expect people to be judged according only to their medical needs. As discussed later (chapter 10) there is uneven access to treatments such as PTCA for people with CHD, and this is one of the priorities that need to be addressed within the UK health service.

Coronary artery bypass graft surgery (CABG)

Coronary artery bypass grafting is a major surgical procedure, yet now done so commonly that patients often stay only a few days in hospital. It is also an extremely successful operation – the majority of people who have a CABG have complete relief of their angina.

The principle behind the procedure is outlined in figure 9. In order to get blood to the area of heart muscle beyond the obstruction the surgeon connects the artery downstream of the obstruction to a supply of blood from higher up. This is done either by using a vein (removed from the same patient's leg) and connecting the upper end of this vein to the aorta or by diverting an artery that runs along the inside of the chest wall to the heart instead (leaving this artery connected to its source of blood from the circulation within the chest wall). Using a vein or an artery from the same person eliminates the problem of rejection that would occur if one tried to use a blood vessel from another person inside the body of the patient.

Figure 9: Coronary artery bypass grafts. (Both vein and artery grafts are illustrated)

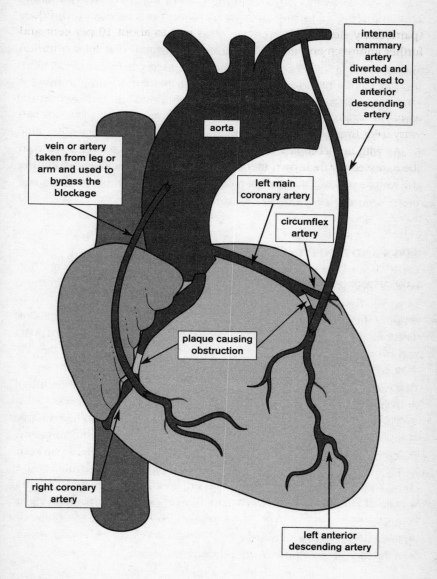

internal mammary artery diverted and attached to anterior descending artery

aorta

vein or artery taken from leg or arm and used to bypass the blockage

left main coronary artery

circumflex artery

plaque causing obstruction

right coronary artery

left anterior descending artery

As we have plenty of spare capacity in our veins we don't miss the loss of one from the leg, and in the case of the diverted chest artery (called the internal mammary artery) blood finds its way to the chest wall tissues it normally serves by other channels. It is also possible to take a piece of artery from the forearm and use that as the bypass vessel – having first checked that there are adequate bypass (collateral) arteries so that blood reaches the hand properly thereafter. In this last technique the artery segment is completely removed and used in the same surgical way as a vein graft.

The advantage of using an artery graft is that it is biologically suited to the higher blood pressure that exists in all arteries. Veins are 'low pressure' blood vessels, and although a vein graft can and does take the higher pressures it is subjected to in a CABG, ultimately the artery grafts tend to better resist re-closure years later.

RISKS AND BENEFITS OF CABG

CABG is a major procedure and death occurs in approximately 2 per cent of operations. In looking at that figure one has to bear in mind however that CABG is often done in people with severe angina, in whom other treatments have failed or been inadequate at giving relief. The quality of life gained by someone following a successful CABG can be dramatic.

A successful CABG *increases* the survival rate of people with severe CHD over the following years and is the only form of angina treatment currently proven to improve survival in this group of patients.

The risk of CABG relates in large measure to a number of identifiable factors. By selecting people at lower risk the outcome of the surgery is much more likely to be successful. This is true of any form of surgery.

Factors which make CABG significantly *more* risky include:

- Age of patient: people over 75 are five times more at risk than those under 55
- Presence of kidney failure
- A history of previous CABG procedure

- Presence of poor heart muscle pumping strength (heart failure)
- Presence of other evidence of atherosclerosis
- Diabetes
- Having all three main heart vessels affected by CHD

Improvements in surgical techniques and in the medical management of angina in general are, however, leading to improvements in results (for both CABG and PTCA) and it is important to realise that angina is not only a highly treatable condition but that for the majority of people affected by it the outcome is very good.

It is now time to bring together the information presented thus far and show how, in an individual with angina, the most appropriate line of treatment is decided upon.

Chapter 8

Deciding the Best Treatment

The preceding chapters have set the scene concerning angina, from the initial development of chest pains and the need to ensure a correct diagnosis, through the associated risk factors that contribute to the development of CHD, and listing the various medical and surgical options available for treatment.

It should have been clear that the diagnosis is not always straightforward and that, even when angina is confirmed, there are many possible ways of treating it.

In the past few years several methods have evolved that provide a structured way in which to assess and treat someone with angina and which ensure that the most effective treatment is being given. The following scheme is based mainly on that recommended by the Scottish Intercollegiate Guidelines Network (an expert medical advisory group) for the management of stable angina. Stable angina is, as the name suggests, the pattern of angina in which predictable symptoms related to effort have been present for some time. In the next chapter we deal with other types of angina that follow a more accelerated or otherwise different sort of pattern and which require a different approach.

You may find it helpful to refer back to previous chapters for more detail on the various lifestyle factors and treatments as they crop up in the following sections.

Stage 1: Initial appraisal and 'baseline' treatments

SEVERITY OF ANGINA
Assuming that the cause of someone's symptoms has been confirmed as due to angina, it is helpful to record the severity of the angina at this stage – and, of course, later as one judges the effect of treatment. There are two simple four-point scales in use (the Canadian Cardio-vascular Society and the New York Heart Association grades) but they are pretty similar:

Grade 1 = Angina only on strenuous or prolonged exercise. No symptoms on ordinary activities.
Grade 2 = Slight limitation on ordinary activity, such as a brisk walk up stairs or into a wind.
Grade 3 = Marked limitation on normal activities such as walking up stairs at normal pace. No symptoms at rest.
Grade 4 = Unable to perform any activity without symptoms, or angina present even at rest.

RISK FACTOR ASSESSMENT
Everyone requires an assessment of their 'risk factors', no matter what the diagnosis, but particularly if CHD has been confirmed as present. To remind you, these are:

- Cigarette smoking
- High blood pressure
- High blood cholesterol

- Family history of coronary heart disease
- Diabetes
- Evidence of 'hardening of the arteries' (atherosclerosis) elsewhere in the body

LIFESTYLE ADVICE AND TARGETS

Figure 10 summarises the various points that should be addressed, and the targets to aim for. These apply to everyone with angina, whatever the degree. We have already touched on each of the main risk factors and what to do about them. It is important to remember that in CHD the risks multiply each other's importance, so if you can chip away a bit at a time from each of the risks that apply to you, you will do yourself a lot of good. Remember you can check your own diet pattern using the list in appendix D. In fact, it is not a bad idea at this stage to work your way down the list in figure 10 and see how you measure up in terms of each risk factor. Do you know your blood pressure, cholesterol level, blood sugar or body mass index, for example? There is no reason why you should not have that information, or at least check that your doctor does. How much exercise do you presently take? How much alcohol do you drink? Do you smoke?

You really don't need a doctor or nurse to tell you if you've got work to do in this area, so you might as well get started!

On first discovering that you might have angina you might be surprised, taken aback and perhaps even a bit frightened – but try to keep it in proportion. The outlook for the majority of people with angina is good, and can be improved by following the sorts of advice in this book and taking the medical advice you are given. You can't immediately rush through a list of risk factors, turning yourself overnight into a different person, but with the right attitude and a determination to get as well as you can, then over the course of a few months it should be possible for you to make a substantial improvement in your present condition and long-term outlook.

Perhaps one of the most important points to emphasise is the need to *go to your doctor* if you begin to get symptoms suggesting angina.

Figure 10: Managing angina (1) – baseline assessment and treatment

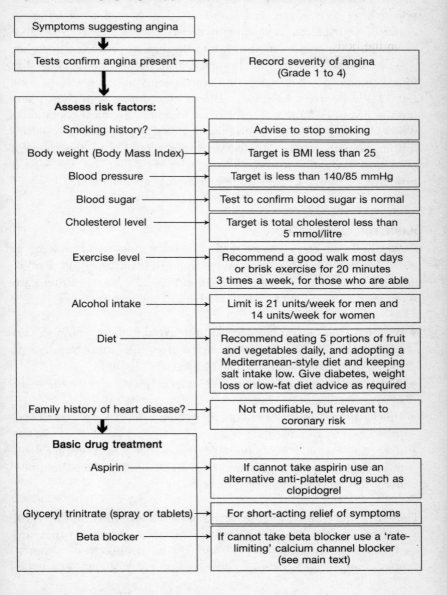

Angina is at its most 'risky' phase in the early days and weeks after it appears, so don't waste time wondering if it is angina, or trying to convince yourself that it is something else.

Of course, it could well turn out to be another problem altogether – as we said at the start of the book there are plenty of conditions that look like angina – but that's not a conclusion you can reach on your own. Many people who present late to their doctor with chest pains (and, it has to be said, a host of other important medical conditions) worry that they will be 'wasting the doctor's time'. Nothing could be further from the truth. No decent doctor would have the slightest hesitation in wanting to see someone with chest pain and to assess it properly – so there's no excuse to delay that appointment.

BASIC DRUG TREATMENT

Generalisations are all very well, but once one starts looking at individual people it becomes increasingly difficult to say in a book like this what ought to happen in an individual's care, but there are some points upon which pretty much all of the experts agree.

- Assuming the person has no reason to avoid it, then aspirin should be prescribed to all people with angina. If aspirin cannot be tolerated then clopidogrel should be used instead.
- A short-acting nitrate, such as GTN (glyceryl trinitrate) for the relief of symptoms, can be started.
- Unless there is any reason to avoid it, then a beta blocker should be prescribed to all patients.
- If, for any reason, it is not possible to prescribe a beta blocker to an individual, then a 'rate limiting' calcium channel blocker should be used instead (verapamil or diltiazem).

These first steps in the treatment process are also shown in figure 10.

Concerning the use of GTN sprays or tablets, although they are useful and quick-acting they should not be needed very often. If someone with angina needs to take several puffs of GTN every day it is likely that their overall treatment is inadequate and needs to be adjusted, so it can be useful to keep a note of how often it is necessary to take a dose of GTN and let your doctor know. If there is a noticeable increase in symptoms, requiring more frequent doses of GTN, this could mean that the angina is becoming more 'unstable'. This should be taken seriously and reported to your doctor, as it might mean that the degree of narrowing in one of the coronary arteries is increasing quite rapidly. That often will be best treated by a hospital admission or at least will need rapid assessment by a heart specialist.

SEEING A SPECIALIST

Up until this stage of assessing and treating angina your own GP is well able to advise you correctly, and will quite probably have also engaged other people in the practice team, such as the nurse and dietician, if you need them. However, it is now considered good practice for the vast majority of people who develop angina also to be assessed by a consultant cardiologist.

For someone with mild angina, well managed with the basic treatment we've already outlined, it might not mean that any further action is required, and your GP can continue to monitor and advise you appropriately. At the other end of the spectrum a very frail or otherwise disabled person who would be unable to cope with exercise tests or coronary angiograms, for example, would not necessarily gain any great benefit from seeing the cardiologist, as the treatment options for that person might be too limited by factors that had little to do with their heart.

We also have to live with the fact that in the UK we have relatively few cardiologists for the size of the problem in the population, and that the distribution of cardiology services is uneven across the country. By applying some basic guidelines such as are summarised here it should be possible to ensure that people who need to be seen by a cardiologist do receive that care. Rapid access chest pain clinics are another way of ensuring that people with recent onset chest pain are assessed in a timely manner. At this stage therefore, with the exceptions above, someone with angina should be referred to a specialist.

Stage 2: Second line drugs and treatment

If symptom relief is inadequate with the first stage treatment then one adds a drug from another group. It is possible for your GP to do this – it would not have to wait until you've seen the specialist. Exactly what that drug should be needs to be decided individually, but generally speaking if already taking:

- A beta blocker, then add:
  a) a calcium channel blocker (like nifedipine or amlodipine. *Not* verapamil, and use diltiazem only with care.); or
  b) a potassium channel activator (nicorandil); or
  c) a long acting nitrate (like isosorbide).

- Diltiazem or verapamil, then add:
  a) nicorandil; or
  b) a long acting nitrate.

- Other calcium channel blocker (like nifedipine or amlodipine i.e. the 'dihydropyridine' types), or nicorandil, then add:
  a) a long acting nitrate.

Stage 3: 'Risk assessment'

The purpose of this stage is to assess the extent of someone's CHD and therefore their level of risk of further heart trouble. This will decide whether further investigation such as an angiogram is required. Cardiologists often use the term 'risk stratification' for this process.

Provided there is no other reason that might make it difficult to do, then an exercise tolerance test will allow the specialist to pick out those people at higher risk. If the exercise test shows a good result (i.e. no signs of heart muscle distress during exercise) and the person's angina is well controlled on medical treatment, then there is no need for further intervention. Those people who show signs on the exercise test that the heart's blood supply is inadequate under exercise can then go forward for an angiogram.

If an exercise test cannot be done then the other types of scan outlined in chapter 4 can be used instead.

Stage 4: Angiogram

The angiogram outlines the heart's blood vessels, confirms where any blockages are located and allows the specialist to assess if intervention is required. Depending on the particular hospital arrangements the next stage of treatment can then be carried out right away or the patient may need to be transferred to a unit with the necessary facilities – see stage 5.

Stage 5: Revascularisation

This, you may remember, is the jargon term for any technique that opens up or bypasses a blocked artery. Depending on the particular specialist's methods, expertise and availability of back-up it is possible to carry out an angiogram to outline someone's coronary arteries and at the same session to carry out a procedure such as a stent. Carrying out treatments like balloon angioplasty and stenting does, however, require readily available back-up from a cardiac surgical team if major problems develop. Therefore, it may be necessary to limit the first session to only making a diagnosis, and if this reveals a need for further intervention, the patient will then need to go to the nearest main medical centre. The cardiologists in your own area will have their own method of doing things but the general plan is likely to be along these lines and will be fully explained to you if you need this sort of treatment.

ANGIOPLASTY OR BYPASS SURGERY?

The decision on which type of revascularisation procedure is appropriate for an individual is very much a personal one and we can only generalise here. Essentially revascularisation should be done when:

- Symptoms are poorly controlled despite maximum medical therapy.
- Assessment by exercise testing and angiography indicates a high-risk situation.

CABG is a bigger undertaking than angioplasty, but improves the outlook for people with advanced coronary artery disease. Indicators that point to a high risk, and that would therefore tend to suggest that CABG is a better option, are:

- More than 50 per cent narrowing of the left main coronary artery.
- Significant narrowing of all three coronary arteries.
- Poor pump action of the left ventricle, secondary to impaired blood flow.

None of these pointers is set in stone. People may have more extensive coronary disease than this and still not be suitable for CABG for many other reasons. Limiting factors might be obesity, lung disease, kidney failure and extensive atherosclerosis elsewhere. Smokers who fail to give up smoking also do badly after CABG, and if someone is not motivated to stop smoking it may not be sensible to proceed to surgery. It is important that you discuss your particular situation with the specialist and with your GP so that you are clear what your own best options are. Ultimately, of course, you have to make up your own mind on how much treatment you are willing to have, and you can only do that if you have all the facts in front of you. Figure 11 summarises the pathway for deciding upon the best angina management in an individual.

Figure 11: Managing angina (2) – treatment choices

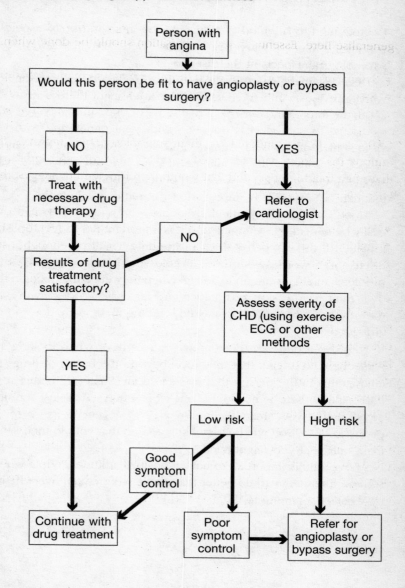

Stage 6: Living with angina

Doctors tend to be good at managing the 'nuts and bolts' aspects of conditions like coronary heart disease but a bit less good at the psychological aspects of the disease.

Developing angina can come as quite a blow, especially to someone with a previously unmarked medical record. Initially there is also worry about the future, and perhaps a real sense of one's mortality. It is good to discuss these concerns openly – with your family and with your various medical advisers. Angina can be well treated and the majority of people with angina should be able to lead an active life. CHD should not be regarded as some sort of ticking bomb but as a condition that can be very greatly improved, if not removed altogether.

Mood disturbance, particularly depression and anxiety, can quite easily be generated by angina and it is important not to feel foolish or ashamed if this happens. Much of the time it will be enough just to discuss your worries with those around you, but at other times these problems might mount up to a level when they need treatment in their own right. Depression and anxiety are far easier to deal with when they are brought out and discussed – hiding them away does no one any good.

It is also a duty that doctors and nurses have when looking after someone with angina that they look beyond the basics of drugs and angiograms to the person that it is all about. Some are better at this than others, there is no doubt, but more often it will just require a mention that you aren't feeling so well in a general sense for the penny to drop. You will be very likely to find that you do then get the extra help that you might need.

Above all it is important to have a positive attitude. People who do so have a tendency to do better than those who remain overwhelmed by what's happening to them.

Chapter 9

Special Types of Angina – and Heart Attacks

Stable and unstable angina

Almost all of the book so far has dealt with the common type, called 'stable' angina, in which the underlying process is usually the slow build-up of plaque within the coronary arteries – a process that develops over years. In the 'classic' angina patient (admittedly more common in medical text books than in real life) chest pains on effort develop first only on strenuous activities and then might progressively become more obvious on lesser effort over months or years. In theory it all happens in slow motion with plenty of time for people to react and adapt.

Of course in real life things can happen more unpredictably and over much shorter time scales. A significant proportion of people who suffer a heart attack have no preceding history of angina and this emphasises the need that we all have to look after ourselves as best we can long before any 'warning signs' of disease develop.

Any change in the pattern of someone's angina is potentially significant but in particular the following should be watched out for:

- More frequent or severe episodes of chest pain (or any of the other types of pain that can potentially be from the heart).
- Increase in need for 'relief' medication (e.g. GTN spray) without obvious cause.
- Increase in breathlessness or fatigue.
- Abrupt onset of angina on effort, or at rest.
- Angina at night.

So called 'crescendo angina' is a similar type of situation, the key feature being a rapidly worsening level of symptoms over a short period of time. If any of these patterns of pain develop they can mean that the degree of narrowing of one or more coronary arteries has worsened.

Various theories exist as to why this may occur, but it seems likely that the surface of the plaque becomes unstable, exposing the underlying fatty layer and other tissues within the artery that encourage platelets to stick and more plaque to form at the site. Short of the artery becoming completely blocked this is the same process that occurs in a heart attack, and should be treated with the same degree of urgency.

Unstable or crescendo angina are conditions that merit urgent hospital admission and if you develop this pattern either speak to your GP right away, or dial 999 for an ambulance.

Syndrome X

In this fairly rare type of angina the person has typical symptoms on effort, relieved by rest and by nitrate drugs, and shows abnormalities in the exercise ECG, yet has normal coronary arteries on angiogram.

Beta blocker drugs usually work well and the outlook is good. Exactly what causes Syndrome X is not well understood, but it is probably due to abnormal blood flow within the microscopic blood vessels within the heart.

Somewhat confusingly there is another Syndrome X! It has long been observed that the following heart disease risk factors are commonly found together in a person:

- Overweight
- High lipid levels
- Tendency to diabetes
- High blood pressure

This cluster is also called Syndrome X, or 'metabolic syndrome'. It is possible that the same underlying biological mechanisms that lead to one also cause the other, but that has not been proven. In the meantime we just have to live with this slightly confusing terminology.

Variant angina

This is also called 'Prinzmetal's angina' and is due to spasm of a coronary artery. Arteries are surrounded by a muscular layer and spasm of this muscle causes a temporary partial blockage of the artery, and consequently angina. Most people who have variant angina do, however, also have significant fixed narrowing of one or more coronary arteries and the spasm tends to occur close to this area of permanent narrowing.

Variant angina does not relate to effort, and often occurs at rest – particularly during the night. Calcium channel blockers tend to give good relief but the overall treatment also depends on the condition of the coronary arteries in general.

Heart attack

A heart attack occurs when a coronary artery, or branch of one, becomes completely blocked and the collateral circulation is insufficient to get blood to the affected area of the heart. A number of consequences can then result. If a large area is affected then the pumping action of the heart will fall significantly, causing a drop in blood pressure and poor delivery of blood to other tissues. The electrical activity of the heart can become unstable, potentially triggering a number of dangerous disturbances of heart rhythm. The most serious of these is 'ventricular fibrillation' in which the regular beating of the heart becomes chaotic and uncoordinated. Unless treated rapidly by an electrical shock from a 'defibrillator' this rhythm disturbance is always fatal. Thirty per cent of people who die from a heart attack do so within the first two hours, usually because of these rhythm problems.

Even if such serious complications do not happen, heart muscle becomes irreversibly damaged after about 45 minutes of being starved of oxygen.

Speed therefore is of the essence – many people still wait too long to call for help following the onset of chest pain. The first response of anyone who thinks they might be having a heart attack is to dial 999 and request an ambulance.

CAUSES AND TREATMENTS

The commonest mechanism behind a heart attack is clot formation, as previously described. Understanding this process led to the development of 'clot-busting' drugs, which, if given quickly enough, can reverse the obstruction and even prevent permanent heart damage.

As aspirin provides some protection against clot development, a very useful 'first aid' treatment that can be done by someone with severe chest pain is to chew an aspirin tablet right away, while waiting for the ambulance to arrive (whether or not aspirin is already being taken regularly).

In hospital the emphasis is on quickly making an accurate diagnosis and on relieving the symptoms such as the chest pain itself. It is not always easy to be certain that a heart attack is occurring but a combination of clinical assessment, ECG findings and blood tests usually make the diagnosis clear. Pain relief takes the form of an injection of diamorphine (heroin).

A drug to dissolve any clot within the coronary arteries is then given through a drip – in the UK this is usually streptokinase. The quicker this is given the better – the so-called 'door to needle time' needs to be as short as possible. The best results from clot-dissolving treatment (properly called 'thrombolytic' therapy) are seen within 6 hours of the start of a heart attack and are uncertain after 12 hours. In some remote areas the problem of quickly delivering a clot-dissolving drug has been tackled by training ambulance paramedics to administer the drug at home. (Ambulance crews also give oxygen from the start and are equipped with sophisticated defibrillators that monitor the patient's heart rhythm continuously.) There can be some difficulty deciding exactly when a heart attack properly started if the chest pain has been intermittent before becoming severe – this is important when deciding if too much time has gone by to make thrombolytic treatment worthwhile; as always, it is best to call for medical help early rather than late.

Thrombolytic drugs do have their disadvantages, particularly as they increase the likelihood of bleeding elsewhere in the body. They cannot, therefore, be given to people who have had a recent operation or other problem that will be made worse by potential bleeding. Even when such people have been excluded there is a risk of complications such as stroke occurring after thrombolysis. The balance of risk is, however, in favour of using the drugs in heart attacks.

There are other techniques available to treat the suddenly blocked coronary artery, including immediate balloon angioplasty. This requires a high degree of skill and access to facilities that it is impossible to provide nationally, so as yet it is not a widely used form of treatment. Research is, however, being done on the best way to combine these different techniques so that those patients most likely to benefit from early angioplasty are treated in this way.

LIFE AFTER A HEART ATTACK

Surviving a heart attack is, for anyone, the first step in coming to terms with an event that has a major impact on every aspect of life. Encouraging someone to regain their physical and mental well-being is the aim of cardiac rehabilitation. It is a process that involves the patient, his or her family and a number of health care professionals.

Participation in an effective cardiac rehabilitation programme reduces the frequency of angina attacks, the amount of medication required, the likelihood of requiring re-admission to hospital and the degree of anxiety and depression experienced by patients. It also reduces overall mortality by around 25 per cent.

There are many ways in which cardiac rehabilitation programmes can be structured and these need not be the same around the country. What is important is that they exist at all and that everyone who has had a heart attack is offered the opportunity to benefit from one.

The Heart Manual is a widely used programme based on a workbook and audio tapes; it can be used by patients in collaboration with a facilitator such as a nurse or health visitor. Details of this and other useful information on cardiac rehabilitation can be seen at http://www.cardiacrehabilitation.org.uk/

Chapter 10

The Challenge of Coronary Heart Disease

The majority of this book has been directed at the management of angina caused by CHD. The measures one can then take to reduce the risk of worsening of CHD are collectively known as 'secondary prevention'. Primary prevention refers to the task of stopping the development of CHD in the first place, in people who have no signs or symptoms of the condition.

Many medical advances have been made over the past ten to twenty years, which have clearly shown that both primary and secondary prevention is possible and effective. With this knowledge have come other major issues that we need to consider at the same time – to do with access to care, costs, resources and our way of living in general.

In these final pages we touch on some of the issues with the purpose of highlighting them. Many or most members of the general public are unaware of the dilemmas and concerns that surround CHD and the other major public health problems that we face today, such as diabetes and high blood pressure. These are conditions that we know we are doing badly at tackling. Many people have these problems and remain undiagnosed for years, with resulting poor health that is at least partly avoidable. Public health policies are established to deal with them (or not) with little reference to the thoughts or opinions of the population they serve. In part that is how we want it – we trust our experts to advise us on the best course of action. However, we live in a world in which decisions are not always made on purely medical grounds alone.

The costs of detecting CHD before it shows up or, preferably, preventing it developing, are staggering. We have nothing like the necessary funds or manpower to do the job properly – not something that governments of any persuasion have historically been brave enough to admit. But that does not mean that we cannot try hard and do the best we can. Nor does it mean that the only way we can prevent CHD is to have every adult with a slightly raised cholesterol level taking a statin drug for decades. There has to be a better long-term solution that has much more to do with our basic diet and exercise level, the avoidance of obesity and the eventual elimination of the smoking habit.

To do justice to this subject would require a book in itself – we have chosen only two issues to highlight. We don't have the answers here, nor do we try to provide them. That is a task that only wider public debate can take on.

Access to care

That the world is divided into the 'haves' and the 'have nots' is clear enough, but such divisions are just as prevalent within the UK. Thirty years ago Dr Julian Tudor Hart, a well-known GP and heart specialist, pointed out that 'the availability of good medical care tends to vary inversely with the need for it in the population served'. We have moved on since then, but perhaps not by much. A 1997 study in Sheffield showed that whereas in the ten most affluent areas surveyed 11 per cent of the population who had symptoms of angina had received revascularisation treatment, only 4 per cent of those in the most deprived areas had been so treated. This survey looked only at the use of NHS facilities so, adding the likely fact that many more affluent people would have had private treatment and therefore would not have shown in these figures, the difference between rich and poor is even more striking.

The reasons for such inequality are many and complex. Many people from deprived backgrounds have low expectations of what they feel they should receive, and too often this is exactly what they get.

Costs and priorities

The ability of statin drugs to lower blood cholesterol level and improve the outlook for people with CHD has been mentioned several times. Their benefit in secondary CHD prevention is undisputed and in primary CHD prevention they have been clearly shown to benefit people with a medium to high risk of developing CHD.

One of the main problems that arises from the use of statins is that they are expensive – about £1 a day at average dosage levels. In England in 1999, 8 million prescriptions were written for statins, costing £256 million. In 2001 the number of prescriptions had risen to 13.5 million, costing £439 million. The Wanless report on the National Health Service predicts that expenditure on this group of drugs alone could be £2 billion annually by 2010.

Faced with such sums that are well beyond any current level of budget allocation, there has been much debate among health officials, doctors and health authorities about 'prioritising' expenditure on statins to the most 'at risk' individuals first. At first sight this seems like common sense – if we can't afford to treat everyone then we should target our expenditure. It doesn't take long, however, to expose some serious ethical problems in such policies.

Current guidelines suggest that, in primary prevention of CHD, statins should only be prescribed to people with a 30 per cent or greater risk of developing serious (fatal) CHD disease over the next ten years. The risk is calculated using one of several published tables that take into account a person's medical history, blood pressure, cholesterol level, etc. (see appendix A for references). The main difficulty, however, is that benefit from statins can be shown in people who are significantly less at risk than this, yet effectively they are not to be treated. If this applies to you, then you might wish to reflect upon whether you feel you have been adequately involved in the decision-making process that arrived at this recommendation.

Summary

Coronary heart disease is a complex subject, difficult to understand and yet extremely important to all of us. It has a fair chance of affecting everyone directly, and for many people reading this book, it already has done so. It is essential that we get to grips with it – from the level of the chemistry of the individual cells in our bodies to the broad sweep of its effect upon the population in general.

Angina is a common result of CHD. It can be serious and disabling but more often it is treatable and tolerable. There is much you can do to help yourself if you have angina. In fact, for all but the most seriously affected people the main treatment will be not with drugs or high technology medical techniques, but with a sensible approach to healthy living, assisted by modern medicine along the way.

No matter how hard one tries though, CHD needs to be actively treated in a significant number of people. The means of doing this have developed remarkably over the past 20 years, and we can now safely carry out procedures that make a significant improvement in the quality of life of the majority of people with angina. It is true that we have a bit of catching up to do to get the best level of care to every section of the community, but by becoming better informed you will help yourself, and others, to overcome this important modern health issue. Hopefully this book will help you in that process.

Appendix A

References

Facts & figures

1 British Heart Foundation statistics: http://www.dphpc.ox.ac.uk/bhfhprg/stats/2000/2002/keyfacts/index.html

Standards of care

1 National Service Framework for coronary heart disease: http://www.doh.gov.uk/nsf/coronary.htm
2 Scottish Intercollegiate Guidelines Network (SIGN), 'Management of stable angina: A national clinical guideline'; http://www.sign.ac.uk/guidelines/fulltext/51/index.html
3 Tudor, Hart J., 'The inverse care law' (Lancet, 1971; 405–12).
4 Payne, N., and Saul, C., 'Variations in the use of cardiology services in a health authority: Comparison of coronary artery revascularisation

rates with prevalence of angina and coronary mortality' (British Medical Journal, 1997; 314:257); http://bmj.com/cgi/content/full/314/7076/257

5 Tod, A.M., et al., 'Barriers to uptake of services for coronary heart disease: Qualitative study' (British Medical Journal, 2001; 323:214); http://bmj.com/cgi/content/full/323/7306/214

Lipids

1 'Prevention of coronary heart disease in clinical practice: Recommendations of the second joint task force of European and other societies on coronary prevention' (European Heart Journal, 1998; 19:1434–503).

2 Primatesta, P., and Poulter, N., 'Lipid concentrations and the use of lipid lowering drugs: Evidence from a national cross sectional survey' (British Medical Journal, 2000; 321:1322–25); http://bmj.com/cgi/content/full/321/7272/1322

3 'Randomised trial of cholesterol lowering in 4444 patients with coronary heart disease: The Scandinavian Simvastatin Survival Study (4S)' (Lancet, 1994; 344(8934):1383–9); http://www.ncbi.nlm.nih.gov/entrez/query.fcgi?cmd=Retrieve&db=PubMed&list_uids=7968073&dopt=Abstract

4 Shepherd, D., et al., 'Prevention of coronary heart disease with pravastatin in men with hypercholesterolemia' (New England Journal of Medicine, 1995, 333:1301–1308); http://content.nejm.org/cgi/content/abstract/333/20/1301?ijkey=kc5tGU6OGlLa2

Smoking

1 Doll, R., 'Mortality in relation to smoking: 40 years' observations on male British doctors' (British Medical Journal, 1994; 309:901–11); http://bmj.com/cgi/content/full/309/6959/901

Diabetes

1 Turner, R.C., et al., 'Risk factors for coronary artery disease in non-insulin dependent diabetes mellitus: United Kingdom Prospective Diabetes Study' (British Medical Journal, 1998; 316:823–8); http://bmj.com/cgi/content/full/316/7134/823

2 Khaw, K.T., et al., 'Glycated haemoglobin, diabetes and mortality in men in Norfolk: Cohort of European Prospective Investigation of Cancer and Nutrition (EPIC-Norfolk)' (British Medical Journal, 2001; 15–18); http://bmj.com/cgi/content/full/322/7277/15

Diet

1 Tang, J.L., et al., 'Systematic review of dietary intervention trials to lower blood total cholesterol in free-living subjects' (British Medical Journal, 1998; 316:1213–20); http://bmj.com/cgi/content/full/316/7139/1213

2 De Lorgeril, M., et al., 'Mediterranean alpha-linolenic acid-rich diet in secondary prevention of coronary heart disease' (Lancet, 1994; 343:1454–59); http://www.ncbi.nlm.nih.gov/entrez/query.fcgi?cmd=Retrieve&db=PubMed&list_uids=7911176&dopt=Abstract

3 Burr, M.L., et al., 'Effects of changes in fat, fish, and fibre intakes on death and myocardial reinfarction: Diet and reinfarction trial (DART)' (Lancet, 1989; Sep 30; 2(8666):757–61); http://www.ncbi.nlm.nih.gov/entrez/query.fcgi?cmd=Retrieve&db=PubMed&list_uids=2571009&dopt=Abstract

Coronary risk

1 Kannell, W.B., 'Hypertension: Physiopathology and treatment' (McGraw Hill, New York, 1977).

2 McManus, R.J., et al., 'Comparison of estimates and calculations of risk of coronary heart disease by doctors and nurses using different calculations tools in general practice: Cross sectional study' (British

Medical Journal, 2002; 324:459–64); http://bmj.com/cgi/content/full/324/7335/459

3 Wallis, E.J., et al., 'Coronary and cardiovascular risk estimation for primary prevention: Validation of a new Sheffield table in the 1995 Scottish health survey population' (British Medical Journal, 2000; 320:671–76); http://bmj.com/cgi/reprint/320/7236/671

4 Joint British societies' coronary risk prediction chart; http://www.hyp.ac.uk/bhs/riskview.htm

Angioplasty

1 Bucher, H.C., et al., 'Percutaneous transluminal coronary angioplasty versus medical treatment for non-acute coronary heart disease: Meta analysis of randomised controlled trials' (British Medical Journal, 2000; 321:73-77); http://bmj.com/cgi/content/full/321/7253/73

Exercise ECG tests

1 Gibbons, L., et al., 'The safety of maximal exercise testing' (Circulation, 1989; 80:846–52); http://circ.ahajournals.org/cgi/content/abstract/80/4/846

Rehabilitation

1 Lewin, B., et al., 'A self-help post myocardial infarction rehabilitation package – The Heart Manual: Effects on psychological adjustment, hospitalisation and GP consultation' (Lancet, 1992; 339:1036–40).

2 Scottish Intercollegiate Guidelines Network (SIGN), 'Cardiac rehabilitation'; http://www.sign.ac.uk/guidelines/fulltext/57/index.html

Appendix B

Anti-anginal Drugs – Class Examples

Only brief details of each drug are given here. Full details are included in the manufacturer's data sheets and can also be viewed within the medicines section of the NetDoctor website: http://www.netdoctor.co.uk/medicines/

The information is accurate at the time of writing but new information on medicines appears regularly. A health professional should always be consulted concerning the prescription and use of medicines.

Medicines and their possible side effects can affect individual people in different ways. The following lists some of the side effects that are known to be associated with these medicines. Side effects other than those listed may exist.

Nitrates – isosorbide mononitrate

HOW DOES IT WORK?

Nitrates release a chemical (nitric oxide) that is made naturally by the body. The effect of nitric oxide on veins and arteries is to relax and widen them, as a consequence of which more blood is supplied to heart muscle and the heart's workload is decreased. As a result, the heart uses less energy, and the pain of angina is quickly relieved.

Tablets and capsules are taken regularly each day to help give 24-hour protection against angina attacks.

DEVELOPMENT OF TOLERANCE TO LONG-ACTING NITRATE

Nitrates can become less effective with time because the body adapts to the medicine and becomes less sensitive to it. When this happens the body can be 'resensitised' by allowing a long gap between doses overnight. For example, a twice-daily dose could be taken at 8 a.m. and 2 p.m. instead of at 8 a.m. and 8 p.m. You should of course check with your doctor before changing your treatment schedule.

MAIN SIDE EFFECTS

- Headache
- Dizziness or loss of balance
- Increased blood flow to the skin on the face (facial flushing)

HOW CAN THIS MEDICINE AFFECT OTHER MEDICINES?

- Sildenafil (Viagra) should not be used with nitrates as this combination causes a large decrease in blood pressure.
- The likelihood of lowered blood pressure or fainting attacks is increased when also taking other drugs to lower high blood pressure.

OTHER MEDICINES CONTAINING THE SAME ACTIVE INGREDIENTS
Chemydur 60XL, Elantan, Elantan LA, Imdur, Isib 60XL, Ismo, Ismo Retard, Isotard, Isotrate, MCR 50, Modisal XL, Monit, Monit SR, Monomax SR, Monosorb XL 60

OTHER NITRATES
- Isosorbide dinitrate is identical to the mononitrate in its method of action and possible side effects.
- Glyceryl trinitrate is commonly used in tablet or spray form for quick relief of angina. It has the same possible side effects, and in view of its quick action can cause more profound attacks of low blood pressure or fainting, particularly when first getting used to the drug. Tolerance to short-acting nitrates such as glyceryl trinitrate does not occur.

Beta blocker – atenolol

HOW DOES IT WORK?
Atenolol belongs to a group of medicines called beta blockers. These block the action of two chemicals called noradrenaline and adrenaline that occur naturally in the body

Their action on the heart causes it to beat more slowly and with less force. The heart therefore uses less energy and the pain of angina is prevented. Abnormal heart rhythms are also prevented or reduced. Due to the reduced heart pumping action the pressure at which blood is pumped out of the heart to the rest of the body is reduced.

MAIN SIDE EFFECTS
- Headache
- Slow pulse
- Dry mouth
- Changes in mood
- Fatigue

- Digestive upset such as diarrhoea, constipation, nausea, vomiting or abdominal pain
- Dizziness
- Wheeze or breathlessness due to narrowing of the airways
- Dizziness on standing due to a temporary fall in blood pressure
- Spasm of the blood vessels of fingers and toes and cold extremities
- Cramping pain in the leg (calf) muscles on exertion
- Rash

OTHER MEDICINES CONTAINING THE SAME ACTIVE INGREDIENTS
Tenormin 25 Tablets, Tenormin LS Tablets, Tenormin Syrup, Tenormin Tablets

Calcium channel blockers – (1) amlodipine

HOW DOES IT WORK?
Amlodipine belongs to a group of medicines called calcium channel blockers. These dilate the blood vessels in the body and are used to treat high blood pressure and angina.

Amlodipine slows the movement of calcium through muscle cells in the walls of blood vessels. Calcium is required for these muscle cells to contract, thus amlodipine causes the muscle cells to relax. This causes the blood vessels to dilate.

Blood pressure depends on the force with which the heart pumps the blood, and on the diameter of blood vessels and the volume of blood in circulation. Blood pressure increases if the blood vessels are narrow or if the volume is high. Dilating the blood vessels in the extremities therefore decreases blood pressure.

The coronary arteries in the heart are also dilated by amlodipine, and this allows more blood, and therefore oxygen, to be delivered to the heart at any time. Overall the heart is required to use less effort to pump blood around the body, and is also given a greater oxygen supply. This prevents the pain of angina, which would normally be brought on because of a lack of oxygen supply to the heart.

MAIN SIDE EFFECTS

- Headache
- Rash
- Increased blood flow to the skin (flushing)
- Reversible inability of a man to have an erection (impotence)
- Nausea
- Fatigue
- Dizziness
- Fluid retention causing, for example, puffy ankles
- Weakness or loss of strength
- Enlargement of the gums

OTHER MEDICINES CONTAINING THE SAME ACTIVE INGREDIENTS

Istin

Calcium channel blockers – (2) verapamil

HOW DOES IT WORK?

Verapamil's method of action is essentially identical to amlodipine.

POTENTIAL PROBLEMS

- Avoid grapefruit juice while taking this medicine, as it may alter the amount of the medicine in the blood.
- The blood levels of alcohol may be increased by this medicine. This can increase the effects of alcohol and cause blood pressure to drop.

USE WITH CAUTION IN:

- Conditions where there is a defect in the heart's electrical pathways resulting in decreased function of the heart (heart block)
- Heart attack (myocardial infarction)
- Liver disease

- Conditions in which the heart rate is slow or the heart muscle's pumping action is reduced

MAIN SIDE EFFECTS
- Headache
- Constipation
- Increased blood flow to the skin on the face (facial flushing)
- Allergy to active ingredients (hypersensitivity)
- Fatigue
- Ankle swelling
- Nausea and vomiting

HOW CAN THIS MEDICINE AFFECT OTHER MEDICINES?
- Verapamil increases the effect of medicines used to lower blood pressure. When first taken with other blood pressure-lowering medication it may cause a large drop in blood pressure and therefore dizziness.
- The risk of heart failure and a severe drop in blood pressure is increased if verapamil is taken with beta-blockers.
- Verapamil significantly increases the blood levels of digoxin to harmful levels. The dose of digoxin must be reduced if these two medicines are used together.
- Verapamil increases the blood levels and therefore the effects of cyclosporin, carbamazepine, theophylline and quinidine.

OTHER MEDICINES CONTAINING THE SAME ACTIVE INGREDIENTS
Berkatens, Cordilox, Cordilox MR, Ethimil MR, Securon preparations, Univer, Verapress MR, Vertab SR 240

Calcium channel blockers – (3) diltiazem

Diltiazem is another calcium channel blocker with a similar range of side effects to verapamil but with less tendency to reduce the heart's pumping action. It can therefore be used, with caution, in combination with a beta blocker if necessary

As with all medications, no change should be made unless directed to do so by a doctor. Sudden withdrawal of a calcium channel blocker can exacerbate angina.

Potassium channel activator – nicorandil

HOW DOES IT WORK?
Nicorandil belongs to a group of medicines called potassium-channel activators, which increase the passage of electrically charged atoms (ions) within the walls of blood vessels. This causes the blood vessels to widen, which allows the heart to work more easily. It also allows more blood to carry oxygen to the heart, and both these effects prevent the pain of angina.

NOT TO BE USED IN:
- Heart failure
- Low blood pressure (hypotension)

MAIN SIDE EFFECTS
- Headache
- Increased blood flow to the skin on the face (facial flushing)
- Dizziness
- Nausea and vomiting

HOW CAN THIS MEDICINE AFFECT OTHER MEDICINES?

- Nicorandil may increase the effect of some antihypertensive medicines (drugs that decrease blood pressure), causing a further drop in blood pressure.
- Sildenafil (viagra) can significantly lower blood pressure if used with this medicine.

OTHER MEDICINES CONTAINING THE SAME ACTIVE INGREDIENTS

Ikorel

'Statin' type cholesterol-lowering drug: simvastatin

HOW DOES IT WORK?

Simvastatin is one of a group of drugs commonly known as 'statins'. They block the action of the enzyme HMG-CoA reductase, which is involved in the biochemical process within the body that manufactures cholesterol. Statins therefore lower the concentration of cholesterol in the blood. They also reduce the concentration of another type of fat, triglyceride, in the blood.

Statins have an important role in the prevention of heart disease as they reduce the risk of cholesterol being deposited in the major blood vessels of the heart (as well as in other parts of the body).

It is important to follow a diet and exercise regime when taking simvastatin, all of which help lower cholesterol.

MAIN SIDE EFFECTS

- Headache
- Rash
- Disturbances of the gut such as flatulence, diarrhoea, constipation, nausea, vomiting or abdominal pain
- Inflammation of the pancreas
- Hair loss

- Alteration in blood tests of liver function and inflammation of the liver
- Pins and needles in the limbs
- Dizziness
- Low red blood cell count (anaemia)
- Muscle pain, weakness and breakdown (myositis)

HOW CAN THIS MEDICINE AFFECT OTHER MEDICINES?

- There may be an increased risk of muscle damage if simvastatin is taken with any of the following medicines: ciclosporin, fibrates (e.g. gemfibrozil), nicotinic acid, itraconazole, ketoconazole, erythromycin, clarithromycin, HIV protease inhibitors (e.g. nelfinavir), nefazadone.
- The 'blood-thinning' or anti-clotting effect of anticoagulants such as warfarin may be increased when taken with simvastatin. This should be monitored when first starting treatment with simvastatin and when doses are altered.

OTHER MEDICINES CONTAINING THE SAME ACTIVE INGREDIENTS
Zocor Tablets

Appendix C

Support Groups and Useful Information

British Heart Foundation

A major UK charity supporting all aspects of research into cardiovascular disease and providing a wide range of information for the public. The website has numerous helpful articles on all aspects of reducing the risk of heart disease and of staying healthy.

England and Wales
14 Fitzhardinge Street
London W1H 6DH
Tel: 020 7935 0185
Fax: 020 7486 5820

Scotland and Northern Ireland
45a Moray Place
Edinburgh EH3 6BQ
Tel: 0131 225 1067
Fax: 0131 225 3258

Website: www.bhf.org.uk
E-mail: internet@bhf.org.uk

British Cardiac Patients' Association

A national voluntary organisation offering help, support, advice and reassurance to all cardiac patients, their families and carers. It also offers advice on how to prevent heart disease and stay healthy.

Website: www.cardiac-bcpa.co.uk/index.html

The Blood Pressure Association

A forum for individuals whose lives are affected by blood pressure, drawing attention to the importance of high blood pressure and trying to ensure better detection, management and treatment. It is a registered charity.

60 Cranmer Terrace
London SW17 0QS
Tel: 020 8772 4994
Fax : 020 8772 4999
Website: www.bpassoc.org.uk

NHS Direct

The online health information site of the NHS in England and Wales.

Tel: 0845 4647
Website: www.nhsdirect.nhs.uk/

NICE – The National Institute for Clinical Excellence

NICE was established in 1999 as part of the National Health Service (NHS) to provide guidance on the current 'best practice' in medicines, medical devices, diagnostic techniques and procedures, and the clinical management of specific conditions.

Website: www.nice.org.uk

PubMed

The National Library of Medicine's online database of medical journal articles, which is free to search over the internet.

Website: www4.ncbi.nlm.nih.gov/PubMed/

Other useful web pages

www.bhf.org.uk/publications/description_nwp.asp?second level=423&artID=1091
This web page, part of the British Heart Foundation's website, looks at the effect smoking has on your heart.

www.cardiacrehabilitation.org.uk/
Information on heart rehabilitation programmes in the UK.

www.hebs.scot.nhs.uk/smoking/smkpstp.htm
A guide to stopping smoking made easier, from the website for the Health Education Board for Scotland.

www.hebs.scot.nhs.uk/topics/heart/index.htm
Information for patients and carers on a range of health topics, including heart disease.

www.riskscore.org.uk/
An online facility that allows you to estimate your future risk of cardiovascular disease.

Appendix D

Diet Information

Diet is an important factor that can contribute to coronary risk. The main dietary features that raise risk are:

- High intake of saturated (hard) fats, fatty acids, cholesterol and calories
- Low intake of fruit and vegetables (below five portions of fruit and vegetables per day)
- High intake of salt

A healthy diet is one that is:
- Low in fat
- Low in sugar
- Where at least five portions of fruit and vegetables are taken every day
- High in fibre

- Contains pulses, e.g. beans and lentils
- Moderate in cereals, bread and potatoes
- Low in salt

This type of diet is recommended for everyone, not just those with coronary heart disease.

Fats and fatty acids

In the Diet and Reinfarction Trial (DART – see appendix A) a daily intake of fish (or fish oil capsules) resulted in a 29 per cent fall in mortality from all causes in the men who took part. Similarly a Mediterranean-type diet has been shown to have a protective effect both for cardiovascular death and recurrent heart attack in patients with established coronary heart disease. These dietary changes would appear to operate through mechanisms other than just the reduction of blood lipids, probably by reducing the tendency for blood to clot.

Fruit and vegetables

A diet high in fruit, vegetables, nuts and grains has been shown to lead to a significant reduction in further heart-related events in people who have had a heart attack. Consumption of fresh fruit and vegetables should therefore be at least the recommended level of five portions per day.

Antioxidant supplements

Antioxidants are chemical substances that are able to 'mop up' other types of chemical in the body thought to be important in causing damage to cells. These damaging molecules are called 'free radicals'. There are many naturally occurring antioxidants – vitamin E, for example – that are present in many foodstuffs. A large research study (the UK Heart Protection Study) is examining the potential benefits of antioxidant therapy but at present there is no evidence to support the use of vitamin supplements in the prevention of coronary heart disease.

Weight reduction

Weight reduction is important in obese people with coronary heart disease, and prevention of obesity by altered diet and exercise is essential.

The potential benefits of a 10 kilogram weight loss in people who are obese are:

Mortality	• More than 20% fall in total mortality
Blood pressure	• Fall of 10mmHg in the systolic blood pressure • Fall of 20mmHg in the diastolic blood pressure
Diabetes	• Fall of 50% in fasting glucose • More than 30% fall in diabetes related deaths
Lipids	• Fall of 10% in total cholesterol • Fall of 15% in LDL • Fall of 30% in triglyceride • Increase of 8% in HDL

Healthy eating assessment

To check your eating habits and to find out where you can make improvements, work through table 2 and the healthy eating action plan that follows.

Table 2: Healthy eating assessment

For each row, write the number of points appropriate for your usual eating habits in the right-hand column headed 'Your Score'.

Type of food	Points				Your Score
	1	2	3	4	
Milk and dairy products					
How often do you eat full-fat cheese? (One portion = a matchbox-size piece of cheese; also include food made with cheese.)	More than once per day	Once per day	2–6 times per week	Once per week or less	
How often do you eat cottage cheese, yoghurts and/or fromage frais?	More than 5 times per day	4–5 times per day	2–3 times per day	Once per day or less	
What type of milk do you use?	Full fat milk	A variety of types of milk	Semi-skimmed milk	Skimmed milk	
Fats and oils					
What type of spread do you use?	Butter	Reduced fat spread	Low fat spread	None	
How much spread do you use?	A thick layer	A thin layer	A scraping	None	
How often do you use cream, mayonnaise or salad dressing?	More than once per day	Once per day	2–6 times per week	Once per week or less	
Do you grill or fry food?	Fry always	Fry mostly	Fry and grill	Grill always	
How often do you fry food?	More than once per day	Once per day	2–6 times per week	Once per week or less	

	Lard/butter	Vegetable oil	Olive oil	Spray-on oil
What kind of cooking fat/oil do you use?				
How often do you eat pastries, such as an apple pie, a meat pie and a Cornish pasty?	More than once per day	Once per day	3–6 times per week	1–2 times per week or less
Fish				
How often do you eat oily fish?	Rarely	1–3 times per month	Once per week	More than once per week
Fruit, vegetables and pulses				
How many portions of fruit do you eat? (Fruit can be fresh, frozen or tinned – with the latter preferably in fruit juice. A glass of fruit juice or any piece of fruit counts as 1 portion.)	Less than 1 per week	2–6 per week	One per day	At least 2–3 per day
How many portions of vegetables do you eat? (Vegetables can be fresh, frozen or tinned. 2 tablespoons of any vegetable counts as 1 portion.)	Less than 1 per week	2–6 per week	One per day	At least 2–3 per day
How often do you eat pulses, e.g. lentils, dried beans/peas and baked beans? (2 tablespoons of any pulse counts as 1 portion.)	Rarely	Less than once per week	Once per week	More than once per week
Meat and meat products				
How often do you eat red meat?	Every day	3–5 times per week	1–2 times per week	Less than once per week
How often do you eat the skin on chicken or fat on meat?	Always	Usually	Sometimes	Never
How often do you eat bacon, tinned or processed meat, sausages, burgers, sausage rolls or pies?	Every day	3–5 times per week	1–2 times per week	Less than once per week

Type of food	Points				Your Score
	1	2	3	4	
Takeaway meals and meals out					
How often do you eat takeaway meals or have meals out?	More than once per week	Once per week	Less than once per week	Less than once per month	
Bread, cereal and potato					
What type of bread, pasta, crackers, pitta bread, chapatis and/or rice do you eat?	None	White	A mixture of white and wholemeal	Wholemeal or wholegrain	
What type of breakfast cereal do you usually eat?	None	Sugar- or honey-coated, or chocolate-flavoured cereals, e.g. Sugar Puffs	Unsweetened cereals, e.g. Cornflakes and Rice-crispies	Bran, oats or wholewheat, e.g. Weetabix, porridge or bran flakes	
How often do you eat chips or roast potatoes (oven-baked or fried)?	5 or more times per week	3–4 times per week	1–2 times per week	Less than once per week	
How many portions in total of the following do you eat per day: ½ cup of rice or pasta; small bowl of cereal; small potato; slice of bread?	None	1–2 portions per day	3–4 portions per day	5 or more portions per day	
Snacks and sugar					
How often do you eat biscuits, cakes or scones?	More than once per day	Once per day	3–6 times per week	1–2 times per week or less	

	More than once per day	Once per day	3–6 times per week	1–2 times per week or less
How often do you eat crisps?	More than once per day	Once per day	3–6 times per week	1–2 times per week or less
How often do you drink non-diet fizzy juice?	More than once per day	Once per day	3–6 times per week	1–2 times per week or less
How often do you eat sweets, ice-cream or chocolate?	More than once per day	Once per day	3–6 times per week	1–2 times per week or less

Salt

How often do you add salt at the table?	Always	Regularly, i.e. most meals	Sometimes, i.e. some meals	Never
How often do you add salt while cooking?	Always	Regularly	Sometimes	Never

Balanced diet

On average, do you think you eat a balanced diet? (A balanced diet is plenty of fruit, vegetables, bread, cereal and potatoes; some meat, fish and lower fat dairy products; little fatty and sguary foods; and no salt.)	Never	Rarely	Most days	Every day

Healthy eating action plan

1 Look at your answers to all of the questions. The higher the number for any answer, the healthier is that choice.
2 Identify the food groups/areas where you could improve your diet by moving to a healthier choice in that section.
3 Then identify the three areas of your diet that you feel you would like to improve upon. (To start with, target those areas for which you have the lowest scores.)
4 Try to tackle these areas, and one month later assess your progress.
5 If you are in any doubt about what sort of food choices to make or need other advice, ask your doctor to refer you to the dietician in your area.